Cindy Damaris Gomes Lira

# Nursing care for people with Down's Syndrome

Cindy Damaris Gomes Lira

# Nursing care for people with Down's Syndrome

## Individual and equitable care

ScienciaScripts

**Imprint**
Any brand names and product names mentioned in this book are subject to trademark, brand or patent protection and are trademarks or registered trademarks of their respective holders. The use of brand names, product names, common names, trade names, product descriptions etc. even without a particular marking in this work is in no way to be construed to mean that such names may be regarded as unrestricted in respect of trademark and brand protection legislation and could thus be used by anyone.

Cover image: www.ingimage.com

This book is a translation from the original published under ISBN 978-620-2-03219-3.

Publisher:
Sciencia Scripts
is a trademark of
Dodo Books Indian Ocean Ltd. and OmniScriptum S.R.L publishing group

120 High Road, East Finchley, London, N2 9ED, United Kingdom
Str. Armeneasca 28/1, office 1, Chisinau MD-2012, Republic of Moldova, Europe
Managing Directors: Ieva Konstantinova, Victoria Ursu
info@omniscriptum.com

Printed at: see last page
**ISBN: 978-620-8-37482-2**

"Without the education of sensibilities, all skills are foolish and meaningless..." (Rubem Alves)

## SUMMARY

This research seeks to investigate which strategies are being used by the nursing team in caring for people with Down Syndrome (DS), and which aspects interact to hinder the success of this care at the Primary Care level. The objectives of this study were to learn about nursing activities aimed at caring for people with DS, to understand the work process of nurses working in primary care and to assess the existence and potential of complementary activities to this approach. The study has a qualitative approach and is based on an in-depth theoretical framework, data collection (through participant observation and semi-structured interviews) and data analysis. The results of the research are discussed in the following categories: professional knowledge about Down's Syndrome; approach to care for diversity in nurses' (in)training; nurses' understanding of Down's in an infantilized way; care for people with Down's Syndrome in health care networks. Based on the discussions, the lack of an academic approach to the care of people with disabilities and DS was pointed out; there was a lack of ongoing training for primary care professionals; there was a lack of human resources needed to meet the dynamics of the service; consequently, care was not singular and disjointed across levels of care, with real transfers of care responsibilities and no sharing of these responsibilities. This reveals the need for care for users with DS to meet the proposals of health promotion, prevention of possible complications and inclusion of these users in society, guiding and applying complementary tools in care (namely, play activities) that enhance the approach of this clientele.

**Keywords:** Down Syndrome, Primary Care, Nursing

# SUMMARY

# 1. INTRODUCTION

Down Syndrome (DS), discovered in 1866 by John Langdon Down, is a genetic alteration characterized by the presence of an extra pair of autosomes 21, i.e. instead of having two chromosomes 21, the individual has three (BRASIL, 2012).

People with DS have particular physiognomic features such as: brachycephaly; a flat face (due to underdeveloped facial bones); a small nose; eyes with an upward lateral slant and epicanthic fold; low-set ears (with narrow ear canals); a small mouth; a tapered thorax; hands with a symphyseal fold and a single palmar fold (BRASIL, [n.d.]). Because of these characteristics, DS is easily identified during nursing consultations, in addition to laboratory analyses carried out during pregnancy, such as cytogenetics and amniocentesis.

Brasil (2012) refers to Down's Syndrome as a public health issue, due to its high incidence rates and possible complications (congenital heart disease, respiratory problems, visual problems, among others) resulting from the anatomical, physiological and cognitive peculiarities that permeate it.

Statistical indicators show that there are more than 300,000 people with DS in Brazil (BRASIL, 2012). Malta (2007) states that by providing appropriate care and guidance that takes into account the particularities of people with DS, deaths can be avoided, i.e. when the susceptibility of people with DS to certain pathologies is addressed, due to their particular physiognomic characteristics, there is a reduction in the cause of death for this clientele. Thus, there is a real need to broaden the understanding of the syndrome by the primary care team, since primary care is considered the gateway to the health care network in force in our country.

According to Brasil (2012), the high rates of people with DS in the country draw attention to the need to review care practices in public health services, especially in primary care. The Basic Health Units (UBS) are important references in health care, working to promote, prevent, rehabilitate and educate in health, through a set of actions that are well articulated with the reality of each individual, taking into account the existing dynamics.

Knowledge about DS in terms of its biopsychosocial aspects is of the utmost importance in health care today. Although it is a subject that receives a great deal of attention from the scientific community, most of the time the findings do not reach the professionals who work in health education units in an appropriate way. This has allowed the Ministry of Health, as the body that articulates policies that promote the protection and recovery of population health, to create Guidelines for the Health Care of People with Down Syndrome, which provide guidance and clarification on diagnosis, treatment and monitoring of people with DS.

However, health care actions should be based on the Expanded Clinic model (which views the individual as a whole), given that this is also the model that guides primary care, as advocated by the Ministry of Health. However, it can be seen that the work of some UBSs is not in line with the recommended guidelines, and most of the time the service is curative in nature, focused on medical care with a biologicist view of the health-disease process, which is not always fully successful (CAMPOS, 2007).

Within the multi-professional care team of these health units is the nurse, who, guided by the guidelines of the Unified Health System (SUS), works in service management, health education practices and direct patient care. According to the principles of equity, universality and comprehensiveness, there should be no restrictions on care, and professionals should be able to adapt to the reality of each user, whether they have a disability or not.

So, in addition to acting on the findings for the diagnosis of the person with DS and the respective outpatient care, the nurse acts to guide the approach to be used by the relatives of the person with DS, always with a positive attitude, demystifying the idea that genetic alterations are limitations to social coexistence.

Brito et al (2009) state that one of the tools used in nursing care is play. They state that the inclusion of playful activities in the nursing care process contributes to humanized care. The use of this tool helps with good communication between professionals and patients, detecting the uniqueness of each one, and is characterized as a resource that aims to facilitate or lead to the objectives set out in the care plan.

According to Viana and Fonterrada (2009), the earlier the person with DS is guided and accompanied in play activities, for example, musicality, play, theatricality; the better their language, thinking, socialization, initiative and self-esteem will develop. These activities influence Down's development as a citizen, making him or her capable of facing challenges and participating in the construction of an egalitarian society. "Through play, human beings express their world of creativity, interacting with themselves and the people around them, in other words, their playfulness goes beyond the barriers of their subjective world" (GIARETTA; ROSA, 2009, p. 481).

Therefore, nursing professionals who are more adept at developing playful strategies as a tool for health education will provide better guidance both in the approach to be used by the family members of people with DS and in the care provided to these clients. Thus, "(...) effective playful interventions for health education should promote learning (evidenced by an increase in the level of knowledge) and broader aspects, such as changing behaviors and improving quality of life" (COSCRATO; PINA E MELO, 2010, p. 263).

People with DS deserve more human-centered care that makes their uniqueness prevail, that sees them as beings with a life, a story, full of needs, desires and longings. This assistance promotes actions that contribute to the integration of people with DS into society. The interest in this research arose from the fact that the national scenario, according to Luiz (2009), presents a large number of cases of DS and from the belief that, due to some anatomical aspects and particular developmental differences, both people with DS and their families need special guidance - indicating the practice of physiotherapeutic activities, occupational therapies, encouraging the inclusion of playful teaching strategies in the daily lives of people with DS, among others. Thus, the nursing care provided must transcend the hegemonic biomedical model of health care, promoting greater integration of these people into society.

We can understand the informative and reflective relevance of this study in the academic sphere (FAEN/UERN), because in addition to being an innovative theme that seeks to articulate playfulness with health care, it enables nursing undergraduates to deepen their knowledge of DS, health education and care for people with disabilities, as well as the care offered to users with DS within the scope of Primary Care.

Thus, this research discusses a topic that is relevant to the training of nurses, contributing significantly to their reflection on the importance of developing policies that provide comprehensive care to all individuals who use health services, especially in primary care, as well as the positive influences of play in caring for people with DS.

Primary Health Care comprises a set of actions to promote health, prevent illnesses, treat and rehabilitate each user, regardless of their particularities. This makes it essential to qualify and reorient health practices, which are currently indicated by the extended clinic model, as advocated by the Ministry of Health.

According to Brasil (2004), the expanded clinic is a model of care that is committed to the individual, viewing them in a unique way. In this model, professionals take responsibility for the users of health services, acting in an intersectoral way, recognizing the limits of individual knowledge, but taking on the commitment to seek out and share other knowledge and skills.

As part of the professional team in this area, nurses, like other professionals, must continually review their work practices, checking that the care they provide matches the demands of each user. Thus, the actions carried out in primary care, represented by the UBS, must be fully implemented and planned. Thus, care for users with DS must meet these proposals, which are: health promotion, prevention of possible complications and inclusion of users with DS in society.

In view of the above, we asked ourselves what strategies and activities are being developed by nurses in caring for people with DS, in order to understand which aspects interact to hinder the success of this care at the Primary Care level, taking as a reference a portion of the care provided in Mossoro.

It is believed that the difficulties faced by professional nurses in providing comprehensive care for people with DS are based on the lack of a specific approach at academic level, which provides adequate knowledge of the main needs of this socially vulnerable group.

One of the other factors that hinder nursing care for people with disabilities is the lack of constant training and continuing education for professionals working in primary care. These professionals, due to the reality of the high demand from their clients and the consequent overload of services, are often unable to provide more singular care to users with DS, disconnected from the other levels of care (MANTOAN, 2006).

On the other hand, the Ministry of Health has come up with alternatives to reverse the reality of care for people with DS who use primary care, developing guiding tools based on the perspective of the expanded clinic in order to strengthen and qualify the service offered in this area. These tools include care guidelines and guidance on encouraging play. As such, the care provided to these users is aimed at preventing clinical problems arising from the peculiarities of the Syndrome, as well as the early cognitive stimulation and inclusion of these people in society.

The overall aim of this research was to find out about nurses' care activities for people with Down's Syndrome in primary care. We believe that this study is relevant to the training and continuity of care in health services, as it has provided us with interesting inputs for discussion, analysis and the proposal of new intervention practices in this area, in a way that has instigated reflection by professionals on the care provided to users with DS, their inclusion in society, as well as their quality of life.

## 1.1 METHODOLOGY

This is an exploratory study with a qualitative approach, and in line with Stake (2011) qualitative research can help a professional to reconsider, during their action, what most needs their attention. A new experience changes intuition; formal/experimental/quantitative knowledge can also do this.

The research areas corresponded to the Basic Health Units (UBS) Marcos Raimundo Costa, Dr. Jose Fernandes de Melo, Dr. Chico Costa, Dr. Ildone Cavalcante de Freitas and Dr. Epitacio da Costa Carvalho, all belonging to the city of Mossoro-RN, and representative of the four health zones (north, south, east and west) of the municipality. The central zone was excluded (because it did not have a UBS with a Family Health Strategy) and the rural zone (due to the difficulty in traveling to rural areas and because it had a different care dynamic from that provided in the urban environment).

In a peculiar way, the study in question also allowed the researcher to encourage the target audience, nurses in primary care, to reflect on the care provided to people with Down syndrome.

The subjects of the study were the nurses working in the Basic Health Units mentioned above. They were invited to take part in the study by means of an invitation letter, which explained the objectives, methodology and ethical principles of the study.

The space in which the interviews took place were rooms in the BHUs themselves, available for use and in conditions of security and confidentiality for the interviewee, with only the interviewee and interviewer present. The reason these professionals were chosen was because they work in the Family Health Strategy (ESF), assisting a considerable number of people, including people with Down's Syndrome.

The inclusion criteria used to select the research subjects were: working at the UBS for at least a year, showing interest in taking part in the research by answering the pre-established questions and agreeing to sign the Free and Informed Consent Form (FICF). The exclusion criteria included: nurses who had been working in the ESF for less than a year, or who were on leave for health or work reasons or on holiday; nursing technicians and assistants.

This research consisted of three stages, the first of which focused on deepening the theoretical framework, when we sought to get closer to the subject. To this end, a literature review was carried out of articles published in journals, books and booklets produced by the Ministry of Health, which mainly discussed care for people with Down's syndrome within the scope of Primary Care. Among the materials evaluated, playfulness was identified as a tool for assisting and guiding people with DS.

"... is a vital part of the research process. It involves locating, analyzing, synthesizing and interpreting previous research (scientific journals, books, conference proceedings, abstracts, etc.) related to your area of study; it is then a detailed bibliographic analysis of the work already published on the subject. The literature review is indispensable not only for defining the problem well, but also for obtaining a precise idea of the current state of knowledge on a given topic, its gaps and the contribution of research to the development of knowledge" (BENTO, 2012, p.01).

The second phase involved data collection, using two strategies: participant observation - in which the researcher got to know the routine of the service and the reality of the areas covered by the UBS, by working directly with the nurses, accompanying them on consultations, home visits, among other activities.

"In the active form of observation, participant observation, the researcher joins the activity as a participant not only to get closer to the other participants, but to try to learn something from the experience they have described on paper. The anthropological pioneer Bronislaw Malinowski was very perceptive about this approach, encouraging us to "leave the camera, notepad and pencil aside and take part in what is happening [...]. Although the degree of success varies, the attempt is possible for everyone" (STAKE, 2011, p.109).

In this way, the speeches presented were based on the actual care situation in these environments, and all the information obtained was recorded in field diaries written by the participating researcher.

Another instrument that provided pertinent inputs for data collection were semi-structured interviews with the nurses involved in the care service, in order to find out more about the care provided to people with Down's Syndrome. These interviews were only carried out after approval by the Research Ethics Committee of Rio Grande do Norte State University (CEP-UERN).

The research was approved with a substantiated opinion coded 722.484, and only after this approval was it continued in accordance with the norms for research involving human beings of the National Health Council (CNS, Resolution **No.** 466, of 12/12/2012), thus respecting ethical issues. After explaining the research to the interviewees, they were asked to sign the Informed Consent Form (ICF).

The names of the participants have been replaced by pseudonyms that connote the qualities and potentialities common to people with DS (caring, cheerful, capable, hyperactive, affectionate, among others), in order to preserve the anonymity of the research subjects and, in a peculiar way, to alter the stigma of powerlessness that descends on people with DS.

In order to record and ensure the veracity of the information obtained during data collection, the interviews will be archived on an mp4 player, which will then be formatted into a pdf file and duly archived. All the materials collected will be kept by the researcher and will be archived for five years.

In the third and final stage, the data collected was subjected to a thorough analysis, combined with field diary records, because according to Minayo (2009), this collection of impressions and notes on the differences between speech, behavior and relationships makes the field research truer, identifying the veracity or falsifiability of the assumptions indicated by the researcher at the beginning of the study.

To analyze the data, we used Bardin's (2010) content analysis, which is a set of communication analysis techniques that seek to obtain indicators that allow us to infer knowledge about the conditions of production/reception of messages through systematic procedures for describing their content. Bardin (2010) states that data analysis is organized into three phases: pre-analysis, exploration of the material and finally, treatment and interpretation of the results obtained.

We have tried to divide the discussion of the research into four chapters followed by a brief final consideration. The first chapter takes an initial look at what Down's Syndrome is, the broad design of the research, the objectives and the methodology used.

The second chapter comprises a theoretical framework, where we contextualize the meaning of intellectual disability, the social construction that permeates Down's Syndrome, as well as counterpoints in the production of health care services - what the SUS has advocated about inclusive care for people with disabilities, and how this has materialized in reality. We also discuss the definition of play and play strategies in the care of people with Down's Syndrome, when we engage in a dialog about play in the lives of human beings and the power play between social classes.

The third chapter refers to the results and discussions, in which the data collected in the interviews is compared to the conceptions of the researchers and of authors who are references in the field of care for people with disabilities. The aim of this research is to encourage the reader to reflect critically on how care for people with disabilities, especially Down's Syndrome, has been configured, and what aspects interact to hinder health care. It also explains the prospects for caring for people with Down's Syndrome in a way that articulates the levels of health care.

Therefore, as one of the intentions, the study brings benefits to those interviewed, enables them to reflect on their practices, highlights their potential and discusses how to tackle the weaknesses in improving the quality of care for people with DS. In this way, this work contributes to the qualification of professionals in training, and likewise of those who work in health services.

# 2 . HISTORICAL AND SOCIAL PROCESS

## 2.1 A BRIEF EPIC OF INTELLECTUAL DISABILITY, WITH AN EMPHASIS ON DOWN SYNDROME.

The manifestations of disability can be classified into three main groups: *physical disability, sensory* disability and *intellectual disability*. Each of them has specific characteristics that are defined by a set of interconnected factors, such as the structure of the disability itself, the person's organic and subjective constitution, as well as their experiences and socio-environmental conditions (DIAS; OLIVEIRA, 2013).

When compared to motor, sensory and communication disabilities, intellectual disability is in a peculiar situation, both because of the inherent invisibility of the individual by a large part of society, and because of the dominant social representations that attribute to people with intellectual disabilities a childish and incapacitating cognition, helping to exclude them from the right to an autonomous and citizen adult life (DIAS; OLIVEIRA, 2013).

Defining disability, particularly intellectual disability, requires an understanding of human complexity. The term intellectual disability has often been associated with madness, which in turn is crossed by negative social representations that still populate the popular imagination today. There is no faithful consensus on the nature of intellectual disability, but its definition is strongly anchored in the medical model, with an organicist orientation, and, sporadically, in the social model (RIZZINI; MENEZES, 2010).

The first studies into disabilities began in the 16th century as part of medicine's concern with classifying individuals who deviated from the standard of normality defined at the time. In the middle of the 19th century, other areas besides medicine, namely pedagogy, came to the fore in discussions and research into intellectual disability (CARNEIRO, 2008).

The terminology intellectual disability has gone through countless conceptual constructions and reconstructions. The French psychiatrist Philippe Pinel used the term idiotism to designate a type of organically-based mental alienation, i.e. a lack of intellectual development; Without much clarity on the predefined concept, one of

Pinel's disciples, Jean Etienne Esquirol, modified the term - from idiotism to idiotia - and characterized the condition by the existence of a generalized and definitive deficit of intelligence, alterations of congenital origin (PACHECO, 2003).

Esquirol apud Santiago (2005) did not consider idiocy to be a disease, but a mental condition, which implied little intellectual development and the impossibility of carrying out "ordinary" activities, such as formal education. Although he sought to distinguish idiocy (amencia) from madness (dementia), Esquirol, Pinel and other psychiatric scholars emphasized a deficient character, which was later distinguished in the conceptual construction of intellectual disability.

During the 20th century, for example, people with disabilities were subjected to "scientific experiments" in Hitler's Nazi Germany. At the same time, without any practical training, they were mutilated in wars, considered heroes in countries like the USA, receiving honors and treatment in government institutions. At the turn of the same century, the ideas of psychiatrist Jaspers Kreapelin - who proposed a system for classifying mental debility as a state of psychic weakness that could lead to varying degrees of mental deterioration - came to the fore in the world of research and analysis of the human being. Mental debility was initially part of a subgroup of so-called chronic psychosis and later came to be considered an incurable degenerative psychosis, characterized by inhibition of psychic development (SANTIAGO, 2005).

In turn, today's more humanistic psychiatric analysis, minimizing the emphasis given to the pathological dimension and the diagnosis of deficit, has highlighted the possibility of education and better social integration of so-called "retarded children" when they are supported by appropriate rehabilitation processes. New educational practices emerged, based on therapeutic objectives and grounded in research and analysis that defended the possibility of reversing idiocy, as well as becoming responsible for understanding mental weakness as an autonomous category, dissociated from psychosis (DIAS; OLIVEIRA, 2013).

It is interesting to follow and understand the historical journey of people with disabilities over time, in order to observe changes in the social perception of this population group, understanding their peculiarities in health care.

People with disabilities, as a rule, were assisted and treated in two ways, looking at Ancient and Medieval history - there is rejection and elimination due to the invalidity and imprecision of the disabled person - and on the other hand, pious welfare protection provided by the Church. In Ancient Rome, both the nobility and the plebs were allowed to sacrifice people born with some kind of disability. Similarly, in Sparta, newborns or adults with some kind of disability were thrown into the sea or over cliffs. In Athens, under the influence of Aristotelian thinking, legal premises were defined which are accepted to this day that "treating unequal people equally constitutes injustice" - a discourse which is now adjectivized as equity. In a way, people with disabilities were supported and accepted from a social perspective, even though they were a minority in society (DEZOTTI, 2011).

The backward way in which people with disabilities were known and treated lasted into the Modern Age, resulting in inadequate, imposing, curative, classificatory and dehumanized assistance and care. In the midst of the Contemporary Age, in the 1858s, people with disabilities (whatever the disability) were included in a group inherent to studies and analysis, along with psychopaths, the alienated and the mentally ill. Such research, worldwide in scope, influenced these specific groups of analysis in Brazil as well.

As a result of an embryonic idea, distorted from the one we have today about disability and people with disabilities, hospices were created to contain and treat the "alienated" and "defective". In Brazil, these welfare measures began when the Society of Surgery and Medicine was established in Rio de Janeiro (DEZOTTI, 2011).

It is important to point out that people with disabilities are a heterogeneous group, bringing together in the same category individuals who may have different motor, sensory, intellectual or multiple conditions. Consequently, health care actions aimed at this segment of the population have to take into account a mosaic of different needs and specificities (BERNARDES et al., 2009).

Biological care, through clinical procedures that quantify disability based on exams and tests, often points to the "disease" and says little about the possibility of the cognitive and social developments present in each person, denying the conceptual breadth that care requires. The reality of nursing care is that many professionals have a generalist view and lack a specific, equitable perspective (DEZOTTI, 2011).

Assisting people with disabilities requires comprehensive and shared care with a view to humanization, autonomy and even the protagonism of the subjects in health practices. It is in this sense that the expanded clinic "(...) seeks to articulate disparate approaches, bringing together different types of knowledge with the aim of guaranteeing the best result in care, by welcoming, dialoguing and involving the subject in the therapeutic process" (BRASIL, 2012).

The expanded clinic links the health system's service network to community resources. It is a transdisciplinary practice and considers the complexity of the individual's life in which the process of illness and social limitations unfolds, as well as care, rehabilitation, prevention and health promotion. It follows a logic of respect and sharing of multiple types of knowledge, dialog, flexibility and responsibility for the service user, whether they have a disability or not (BRASIL, 2012).

In this process of constructing and reconstructing what it means to care and how to care, new guidelines for care conduct were created that significantly changed the way people with disabilities were cared for, when changes in international documentation transformed movements by so-called "minorities" into a progressive recognition of the need for changes in legislation, society and the very recognition of people with disabilities,

Among the documents that legitimize and strengthen the rights of people with disabilities are the "Universal Declaration of Human Rights - UDHR" drawn up by the Brazilian World Organization - UN[1] . In 1975, the General Assembly of the United Nations Organization defined the Declaration of the Rights of Persons with Disabilities[2] . In 1999, an Inter-American Convention for the Elimination of All Forms of Discrimination was organized in Guatemala.
against people with disabilities (SILVA; DESSEN, 2002).

Recognition of the individual with a disability as a discourse today was also consolidated at the International Congress "Inclusive Society" in 2001. Based on this discourse, the Montreal International Declaration was defined - where it is initially

---

1 Signed into law in 1948, it advocates respect for every individual, regardless of religion, color, ethnicity, gender, language or political opinions, and strives for pleasant civil coexistence. Taking the UDHR as a starting point, socio-political organizations have developed other documents and rules of conduct to better guarantee and visualize the rights of people with disabilities.

2 The General Assembly, jointly cooperating with the United Nations Organization, in order to promote better life expectancy, permanent work for all, conditions for progress, economic and social development for people with disabilities, proclaimed the DECLARATION ON THE RIGHTS OF PEOPLE WITH DISABILITIES, which calls for the
the adoption of measures at national and international level for common bases and benchmarks to support and protect the rights of people with disabilities

corroborated that all human beings are born free and are equal in dignity and rights, and from its notes that intergovernmental declarations raised the international voice to bring together governments, workers and civil society in order to develop inclusive policies and practices (SASSAKI; XAVIER, 2001).

All of these legislative milestones and mobilizations were aimed at recognizing the rights of people with disabilities and, without a doubt, people with Down syndrome. Up to the present day, regulations have been organized and produced to support the rights of people with disabilities, recognizing them as citizens, in order to overcome their historically constructed invisibility. The discourse on intellectual disability, concomitant with public policies, is inviting us, from the perspective of changing interpretations, to think about prejudices and conceptions that stigmatize people with intellectual disabilities as useless. It is a current and urgent discourse (SILVA; DESSEN, 2002).

Farias and Buchalla (2005) state that the World Health Organization (WHO), in order to respond to the need to recognize and learn more about the consequences of illnesses and disabilities, published the International Classification of Impairment, Disabilities and Handicaps (ICIDH) in 1976. The document was created with the aim of classifying and understanding the functionality of disabilities, in order to code and quantify the developmental coefficients of people with disabilities.

However, after several versions, the ICDD revision process revealed weaknesses in relation to the dimensions that make it up, such as social and environmental aspects. In May 2001, the World Health Assembly approved the International Classification of Functioning, Disability and Health[3] (ICF). The Portuguese-language version became known as the International Classification of Functioning, Disability and Health (ICF), in order to better classify disabilities, reflecting a better organization of health care (INTERDONATO; GREGUOL, 2012).

According to the World Health Organization (WHO) (2004), in the international classifications of health conditions (diseases, disorders, injuries, etc.) people with intellectual disabilities, as well as Down's Syndrome, are mainly classified in the ICD-10 (abbreviation for the International Classification of Diseases, Tenth

[3] A classification system with the name approved during the 54ª World Health Assembly, known as ICF for short, with a view to its use in different countries. In its official Portuguese version, it was called the *ICF - International Classification of Functioning, Disability and Health.*

Revision), which provides purely biological information.

Functionality and disability associated with health states are classified in the ICF. ICD-10 and ICF are therefore complementary, and their users are encouraged to understand these two classificatory members together. ICD-10 provides a "diagnosis" of diseases, disorders or other health conditions, which is complemented by the additional information provided by the ICF on functionality.

Both classifications (ICD and ICF) use a pattern of letters and numbers in their language in order to unify and standardize the understanding of disability through a classification method. This often labels and delimits the cognitive and intellectual capacity of people with disabilities, generating a concept of incapacity or limitation about them.

In a joint and complementary way, the information on diagnosis and functionality makes it possible to visualize the health of people with disabilities and the population as a whole in a broader and more meaningful way. This analysis undoubtedly helps in decision-making regarding the construction and reconstruction of a health care system. Thus, what is defined as intellectual disability and the notable reduction in cognitive abilities are part of this definition/classification of people with DS.

In ICD-10, DS is given the code Q - 90. As it is classified in the Classification chapter, it defines diagnoses, therapies and the specific characteristics of Down Syndrome care (INTERDONATO; GREGUOL, 2012).

In addition, and beyond pathophysiological research, the ICF describes health-related states, focusing on the components of health and the consequences of becoming ill. Two domains are used as evaluation criteria: the first is Body Function and Structure and the second is Activity and Participation (INTERDONATO; GREGUOL, 2012).

In addition, the ICF relates individual subjective aspects of people with disabilities to the environmental and contextual factors with which they interact, such as family support, personal and community resources, access to health care and others. The ICF can be used as a tool for managing care services in terms of diagnosis, therapeutic proposals and follow-up. However, it also helps to plan public health policies and educational programs.

When the aim is a continuous assessment of clinical follow-up, as is the case with DS - due to its physio-anatomical particularities, it is recommended that the ICF be used in addition to the ICD, which makes a paradigmatic shift from the disease axis to the health axis and makes it possible to understand a person's condition or state of health within a broader and more diverse context (BRASIL, 2012).

The current definition and classification of the term disability has been historically and socially constructed, with the concepts of disability and illness often understood as synonyms. Perhaps for this reason, people with disabilities in many societies have been kept apart from public policies and non-governmental health promotion initiatives (INTERDONATO; GREGUOL, 2012). It is of fundamental importance to understand this defining historical process and, based on this discussion, to understand the perspectives of assisting people with disabilities, especially those with Down's Syndrome, visualizing between the lines assistance activities directed at people with DS at the level of Primary Care.

Through legal and social discussions, the global and national political scene has tried to rearrange itself in a more equitable way, establishing rights and developing measures to care for people with disabilities, albeit in a small way (IBDD, 2008).

Understanding that citizenship is one of the fundamental principles of the democratic state, in other words, anyone who has rights and obligations, protecting their dignity, exercising solidarity and claiming what is due to them, that is being a citizen. The disabled person is a citizen like any other (SOARES apud CARVALHO, 2004). This right must be respected by everyone and in all situations, such as health, education, transportation, work, leisure, access to justice, among others. Ratifying the legal rights of people with disabilities means demanding a guarantee of their respect and autonomy (MELO; FARIA, 2009).

Because Down's Syndrome is an intellectual disability, it also received (and in some cases still receives) dictatorial, biologically-centered, infantilizing care, which does not contribute to the autonomy and social inclusion of the person being cared for. The first forms of care involved isolating the individual in order to control him or her, treating the issue of disability as a disease; care linked to psychiatric ailments with a medicated, restraining nature. Another stance was generally to relate the anomaly to a conjuncture of social, religious, moral, climatic and even economic factors. Depending on these circumstances, characteristics and conveniences, people could be classified in a state of madness, insanity and disability, and thus treated, or rather isolated (DEZOTTI, 2011).

In Brazil in particular, we can say that public policies aimed at assisting people with disabilities are recent. The one that provided the best detail for actions both in the Unified Health System and in the various government bodies, as well as in intersectoral relations and partnerships with non-governmental organizations in society, was that published by the Ministry of Health in Ordinance No. 10.060/2002 (BRASIL, 2006b). This, in turn, according to Farias and Buchalla (2005), emphasizes that it is necessary to "rehabilitate people with disabilities in their functional capacity and human performance in order to contribute to their full inclusion in all spheres of social life" and "protect the health of this segment of the population, That is, by legal means, health services must contribute to the promotion of the social inclusion of people with disabilities, both through information and guidance, as well as through the provision of preventive care for problems common to disability.

The National Health Promotion Policy - PNPS (BRASIL, 2006a) defines health promotion as a "health production" strategy, that is, as a set of articulated actions developed in Brazil's public health system that can contribute to meeting society's health needs. The policy also highlights the need to make architectural and furniture changes in order to guarantee access to health services for people with disabilities, while also stressing the importance of providing opportunities to participate in physical activity programs (INTERDONATO, 2012). This policy is one of the legal protections for assisting people with disabilities, but it does not eliminate the need to re-evaluate how assistance has been provided to these people.

Thus, it is necessary to clarify that the historical path in which people with disabilities were gradually incorporated and considered into the social fabric or structure is an erratic, non-linear process, invariably marked by individual trajectories. It is not possible to visualize a continuous and homogeneous movement of integration, because the feelings and the way in which society viewed people with disabilities varied over the course of historical and social formation.

## 2.2 "SLOW AND SMART, STUPID AND BRILLIANT": SOMEONE MAY THINK THAT ABOUT THEM - DOWN'S SYNDROME, A SOCIAL CONSTRUCTION.

According to the World Health Organization (WHO, 2004, p.18), there are currently two models for understanding disability: the *medical model* and the *social model.* For the medical model, disability is "a problem of the person, caused directly by illness, trauma or other health problem, which requires medical assistance in the form of individual treatment by professionals". The social model understands disability as a social problem that is permanently related to the functionality expressed by the person, i.e. it is "the result of a complex relationship between the individual's health condition and personal factors, with the external factors that represent the circumstances in which the individual lives" (WHO, 2004, p. 15).

Farias *and* Buchalla (2005) state that the term *functionality* refers to the functions and structures of the body, as well as activity and, above all, social participation. It is not something inherent to the individual themselves, but also concerns the current social conditions, which must provide the environment with restructurings that allow the person to be included in the various ambits of social life. Since the promotion of social change is an ideological and political issue, it is up to society to provide adequate means to enable people with disabilities to participate fully in society (WHO, 2004).

In the discussion about intellectual disability, different conceptions emerge that predominantly value the individual dimension to the detriment of the socio-cultural dimension, and highlight the subject's limitations revealed through the testing of intelligence levels, disregarding the development possibilities present with adequate stimulation and social interaction (DIAS; OLIVEIRA, 2013). It is necessary to overcome the stereotype of slowness or mental stupidity by which people with intellectual disabilities are still perceived; to enable social interactions that prove how bright and clever they are.

Understanding disability today requires knowledge of the historical and cultural construction of its concepts, current conceptions and scientific criteria for identifying it. It also requires recognizing how people with disabilities construct notions about themselves and narrate their experiences in dialogical contexts.

With a cultural-theoretical basis, in this subchapter - which refers to the social construction of Down's Syndrome - we will take on ideas and thoughts from Vygotsky, Marx and Engels, appropriating arguments for understanding disability as one of the possible manifestations in the process of human development.

It is necessary to understand intellectual disability from a qualitative and not a quantitative point of view, not just as if the person lacked an ideal coefficient of intelligence, similar to when referring to people with visual or hearing impairments, among others; or as if the person with intellectual disability lacked the very essence of humanity - rationality (PAULA, 1994).

Intellectual disability should not be understood solely as a disability of its own, but also as a condition that develops from the social relationships established with individuals who have significantly different characteristics from the majority of the population. Even in the face of any organic alteration, even at the structural or functional level of the nervous system, it is also through social relationships that the subject will develop.

There are currently projects and programs that diverge from the neurological biologist idea - in which intellectual disability is known as irreducible limitations. These projects affirm and prove that cognitive and learning limitations can be overcome: Saad's work (which focuses on the school learning process of young people with DS), the Lurdinha Program (which points out multiple possibilities for the development of children with DS), the Roma Project (with a multidisciplinary team of teachers, family members and people with disabilities discussing and working on the teaching-learning process of people with DS), among others (CARNEIRO, 2008).

These programs and projects start from the premise that there are cognitive and cultural possibilities for the development of people with intellectual disabilities in order to counter the classic concept of purely innate intelligence. Lopez (2003) states that in order to build a new perspective/theory of intelligence, we cannot continue to maintain the principle of innate and general personal capacities in human beings, as this leaves aside the differences that make us human beings.

Therefore, we are moving towards the understanding that the human being must be seen as a whole, although at least four dimensions are proposed for understanding this whole: cognitive processes, affectivity, autonomy and language as communication.

When we want to improve the cognitive, linguistic, affective and autonomy conditions of people with intellectual disabilities, such as Down's Syndrome, it is necessary to qualify the contexts in which they live. Development is determined by the peculiarities and idiosyncrasies of each individual, as well as by the sociocultural environment in which they live (CARNEIRO, 2008).

Following Vygotsky's (1998) reasoning, man is a thinking being who represents what he does to himself and to others. Man produces and thinks: he produces materially and produces representations, ideas, about his material production. These representations, these ideas form consciousness, which in turn is determined by the material conditions of production. It is through these productions that man relates to other individuals, forming social coexistence.

Human material production requires the aid of instruments, since human activity is instrumental, and these instruments are both physical and psychic in nature (signs, which modify relationships between subjects). Signs are mediators of human activity and, as such, are constitutive of man, i.e. human activity is always mediated by cultural signs that form a symbolic existence (CARNEIRO, 2008).

Symbolic systems, especially language, function as mediating elements that allow communication between individuals, the establishment of meanings shared by a given cultural group, as well as the production of meanings, which make it possible to perceive and interpret the world in which we live (CARNEIRO, 2008). With this in mind, Vygotsky (1998) states that man's mental and intellectual functioning processes are fostered by culture, by symbolic mediation.

At birth, human beings only have the biological resources characteristic of their species, which are considered the basis for the process of humanization. However, it is living with others that will enable this process to take place. From the moment an individual is born, they progressively enter a world where relationships are mediated by the values, meanings and truths of their culture. It is not that the individual will passively be shaped by culture, but that they will interact with it (CARNEIRO, 2008). Therefore, man is both a product and a producer of culture, in other words, we participate as a singular subject in social circumstances, who has been singularized by his culture.

The complex biological-cultural relationship brings us back to the way in which each person appropriates social practices. Vygotsky (1998) clarifies the meaning of the word social in his theoretical propositions, in the broad sense of the word everything that is cultural and social. Culture is precisely the product of social life and the shared activity of men, so the very idea of cultural development already introduces us to the social plane, which is thought out, defined and often inflexible.

It is important to note that in the presence of a disability, it becomes clearer that the development process does not occur naturally, but is triggered by concrete living conditions, which are not pre-defined solely in the individual and the family or cultural group to which they belong, but are built up in social relationships. Based on the meanings initially attributed by others and later internalized by the individual in their own context, each person is constructed in a unique way. From this perspective, we cannot accept the reduction of the subject to some peculiarities present in their developmental trajectory, such as physical, intellectual, hearing or visual disability, among others. Because it is the attribution of meanings to this peculiarity that will build this subject, who will continue to have their organic characteristics, but who will define, always in relation to the other, a unique way of being and being in the world (CARNEIRO, 2008).

However, we know that there is a different hegemonic conception of human development, built in ancient times, but which is reflected in today's society. In the middle of the 19th century, a famous French psychiatrist, Philippe Pinel, in one of his analyses compared a boy with intellectual disabilities to others who lived in an asylum, and concluded that this boy had been abandoned because he was an idiot and there was no possibility of educating him, classifying him as a young savage, unfortunate in intellect, far inferior to some of the domestic animals. Notes like these, even if they are retrograde, still permeate the minds of some individuals who dismiss people with intellectual disabilities as slow and stupid (LEITE; GALVAO, 2000).

Opposing Pinel's diagnosis, Jean Itard at the same time pointed out that man is not born as a man, but is built as a man. He considered the boy's retardation to be not only a biological deficiency, but also a cultural insufficiency, a lack of experiences of intellectual exercise, so the stimulation and ordering of intellectual and social experiences would constitute strategies for "curing" the boy (LEITE; GALVAO, 2000).

However, even if new conceptions of intellectual or mental disability were to emerge, the conceptual genesis of intellectual disability, which is essentially medical, would remain organicist, emphasizing both its genetic or perinatal determination as well as non-encouraging prognoses. As a result of this fatalistic organicist principle, segregation between the so-called "normal" and "disabled" existed and still exists as a way of guaranteeing social order. However, the hegemony of the organicist medical doctrine gradually lost ground and was severely criticized as ideas about the educability of people with disabilities developed and were confirmed, and the concept of incurability returned to intellectual disability began to be worked on and reinterpreted through educability, the integration of people with disabilities into social life (CARNEIRO, 2008).

The aim is not to bring about the acceptance of people with disabilities in society by obligation, but rather to encourage reflection on the countless possibilities and abilities that these people have, and to break down the stigmatization and crystallization of the limiting labels with which people with disabilities, especially intellectual disabilities, are seen.

Among his thoughts and ideologies, Vygotsky (1997) presents a central thesis of defectology, stating that every defect or disability creates stimuli for compensatory development, and that compensatory processes constitute a potential for the development of the disabled person. He also points out that the process of compensation will not always be successful, nor does it occur naturally; it is a process of overcoming and struggle. There is always a reaction to the disability, which triggers compensatory processes, but it must be emphasized that the innate organic causes do not act on their own, but indirectly through the social place the person occupies in the presence of some limitation.

Compensation processes create new pathways for development, for example, a blind or deaf child can reach the same levels of development as a "normal" child, but they do it in a different way, by different means. When what is altered are the natural processes of sight, hearing, movement or intellectual activity, what needs to be developed are the higher processes, through education, care and health guidance appropriate to the particularities of each individual. Therefore, only sensorimotor training, simplified and repetitive activities and pharmacological treatment of complaints do not contribute to the processes of social compensation, or in other words, social development (CARNEIRO, 2008).

When discussing and working with health, it is essential to understand health care beyond the biological curative approach of assessment-diagnosis-treatment-cure. Melero (2004) criticizes the classic concept of diagnosis, which labels people with disabilities as sick, retarded, deficient or subnormal. This concept of diagnosis expresses the deficit paradigm and offers people no possibility of change, a fragmented, static, deterministic and classifying diagnosis. In fact, there is a possibility of change in the form of educational paradigms, of playful stimulation that recognizes people with disabilities as people and not as sick, so that the diagnosis is not limited to deficits, but points to skills to be developed.

Therefore, especially in health care services, it is more important than diagnosing a disability to present proposals for interventions that promote development, which go beyond diagnosis as a threshold of knowledge to an open door for discovery, an invitation to search for new mechanisms and mythologies for development. Human development is not about pointing out what someone is now, but what they can be with educational and cultural help (MELERO, 2004).

Vygotsky (1997) differentiates between primary and secondary aspects of disability. The primary aspects refer to organic, cerebral lesions, congenital malformations, chromosomal alterations, in other words, physical characteristics commonly pointed to as the causes of disabilities; the secondary aspects, on the other hand, reflect the difficulties, including social difficulties, generated by the primary aspects.

"The action of the defect itself is always secondary, not direct, but reflected. The child doesn't feel their disability directly. The direct consequence of the defect is the lowering of the child's social position; the defect is realized as a social deviation." Vygotsky (1997, p.18)

The idea of incompleteness or deficient cognition in children or people with intellectual disabilities is linked to the social relationships established between people with disabilities, their individual difficulties and the environment in which they live.

Intellectual disability as a social production is the result of relationships with the subject who has intellectual cognitive impairment, as well as with subjects who do not have any organic impairment (ROSSI; ROSSI, 2012).

It is not a pretension to deny the existence of mental-intellectual disability as

condition presented by subjects with organic impairment, but rather to understand that this condition is not initially given, but is built up to the extent that development conditions consistent with their peculiarities are not made possible (CARNEIRO, 2008).

Children begin their development in a world that is already humanized, loaded with social meanings and attributes by the generations that belong to it. Since this development is permeated mainly by family interactions and significant experiences of appropriation of cultural values, in the case of children with disabilities these experiences need to be intensified in order to guarantee the possibility of the formation of higher functions, functions that direct a new path of competence, in order to guarantee the same experiences as people without disabilities (CARNEIRO, 2008).

In this sense, for Garcia (1999 *apud* Carneiro 2008), intellectual disability can be understood more as being influenced by the concrete conditions of life, by the relationships that are established between people, rather than by personal characteristics due to organic limitations. Thus, it is possible to understand that people, even those with physical characteristics socially identified as disabled, can relate and constitute themselves in other ways, based on other relationships.

When it comes to social contexts, as long as the subject does not have access to the universe of signs and the processes of signification, they do not develop higher forms of thought. Therefore, this lack of development, the stigma of the intellectually disabled, is more related to the scarcity or even the absence of opportunities for semiotic mediation[4] than to injury or chromosomal alterations or any other organic condition, signified as individual incapacity.

If we consider the organic condition of the person with Down's Syndrome

[4] Interpretation and production of communication signals, relationship between signs and signals in communication (FIDALGO, 1999).

(specific intellectual disability), we know that trisomy 21 alters various cells, all systems, especially the nervous system, both in the formation of structures and in the cognitive-behavioral functional adaptation itself. From this point of view, the possibilities for cognitive development are limited, as there are structural and functional alterations. However, if, in the face of these altered conditions, we provide people with DS with "environmental, social nourishment" with lots of stimuli, challenges and access to the mediating signs that enable the formation of higher functions, it is impossible to predict the limits and possibilities (CANEIRO 2008).

If we start from the premise that every human being can learn, can develop, it becomes logical to say that everyone, even with significantly different physical, mental, sensory, neurological or emotional conditions, can develop higher functions. It is possible to improve the relationship between people with certain limitations, biologically speaking, and those who don't, and it is possible to reaffirm that human development always takes place in the intertwining of biological and cultural aspects.

## 2.3 PRODUCTION OF HEALTH SERVICES: FROM JARGON TO PRACTICE.

"All human beings are equal. All people must be recognized as integral, dignified beings, with the right to physical and moral integrity; they deserve freedom, peace and justice" (BRAZIL, 2009), a very common discourse, a veritable jargon, in social organizations, including in the health care sectors.

Reflections and considerations must be made about this discourse, understanding that as beings everyone is equal, but each person has their own particularities. It is the life stories of each individual and their particular personality traits, which will depend on where they were born, what education and working conditions they have, and in which society they are inserted that differentiate them.

Brasil (2009) reports that citizens must be guaranteed equal opportunities in all life situations, so that they can develop their potential. Health care that is consistent with the demands and needs of the people who make up and build society, including those with disabilities, must be ensured. People with disabilities, whether physical, sensory or intellectual, must be seen and assisted in accordance with their particularities, and encouraged to develop their potential and skills, and not kept to an incurability based exclusively on the biological standard defined as "normality".

As seen above, there are various treaties, projects and plans signed by nations around the world, including under the coordination of the United Nations (UN), which seek to recognize the principles of equality while maintaining respect for differences. They are truly international norms that emphasize the security of rights among citizens (BRASIL, 2009).

While still discussing legal principles and regulations, health, understood as a citizen's right and a duty of the state, needs to be understood as a social policy, i.e. a policy that focuses on the conditions of individuals and the community, assuming health as one of the rights inherent to the condition of citizenship, since the full participation of individuals in political society is achieved through their inclusion as citizens (FLEURY; OUVERNEY, 2013).

Citizenship presupposes the existence of a national political community, in which individuals are included, sharing a system of beliefs with regard to public authorities, society itself and the set of rights and duties attributed to citizens. Belonging to a political community also presupposes a mutable legal and political bond that recreates civic culture, and citizenship itself, at each social historical moment (FLEURY; OUVERNEY, 2013).

Citizenship therefore implies a principle of justice that has a normative function in the organization of the political system, and is contemporary with the development of modern states and the capitalist mode of production. In these states, power is exercised in the name of the citizens, who must legitimize political authority, understood as the democratization of the political system.

However, when we want to design a health policy, we think of objects of sectoral realities, strategies and modifying instruments. Remembering that this policy can affect and be affected by other areas and by other relationships, such as economic, political or cultural relationships. Therefore, we can understand that health policies, their strategies, instruments and plans produce an action that is not limited to the field of health, since, being able to influence various other aspects of social dynamics (economic, political, cultural), they can also fulfill various other roles, or functions, in addition to their basic objective of solving "health problems" (WERNECK; FARIA; CAMPOS, 2009).

Fleury and Ouverney (2013) state that health policies are seen as decision-making processes involving social actors and interests, which take place in institutional and organizational environments through which priorities and strategies are defined that relate the means to the proposed ends, in other words, it is the legitimization of health care based on the reality of each citizen.

When we produce a particular health care or health policy, we need to understand that its elaboration covers a cycle made up of planning, implementation and execution stages, in which various actors take part and must evaluate and shape the general format of the policy according to the time frame, culture and needs of each citizen. Even understanding the complexity of health care, it is necessary to have equity, to adapt care to each reality, to each user of the health service, whether they are disabled or not.

Therefore, like all citizens, people with disabilities should seek out health services when they need guidance, prevention, general or specific care. The professionals working in these services must have the necessary knowledge to provide comprehensive care to each user. It is important that not only do users seek out health institutions, but that the health service reaches out to the user, understanding and considering each particularity, and continuously assessing the general state of health of each individual (BRASIL, 2009).

In general, our health care is organized under a Unified Health System, with a view to anticipating care for health problems or trying to solve them quickly. In this way, the care model has been configured in a dynamic of multidisciplinary, comprehensive and equitable care. It is organized into levels of care, which are guided by care programs and protocols that interact with each other through care networks. The level of care with the greatest contact and monitoring of the population is Basic Health Care - represented by the Basic Health Units, which are guided by the Family Health Strategy (WERNECK; FARIA; CAMPOS, 2009).

The Basic Family Health Units (UBSF) must welcome their users, provide assistance for complaints, advise on complementary tests, supply basic medicines, monitor the progress of each case and refer them to specialized care units when necessary, as well as monitoring those users who do not have complaints, from a preventive perspective with the help of health education practices (FIGUEIREDO, 2011).

The Nucleos de Apoio a Saude da Familia (NASF - Ordinance MS/GM No. 154/2008), which work with a multi-professional team formed according to the characteristics of each municipality, provide treatment and follow-up to users with technical and professional support. This monitoring follows people with disabilities, with a view to identifying them early, working on acceptance of the disabled person, their family members and, above all, the society in which they live, so as to also work towards rehabilitation according to the difficulties encountered (FIGUEIREDO, 2011).

Assessing the family situation and dynamics involves not only the emotional conditions and socio-economic, cultural and educational situations of the individual, but also their expectations regarding the process of rehabilitation, education and professionalization - processes that are strongly influenced by social opinion. Parallel to the rehabilitation work, it is very important for the disabled person and their family to be linked to a UBSF, and not turn to specialized care because of the disability. As a result of the stigma attached to disability, especially intellectual disability, many people with disabilities and even their families do not seek out basic care services, resorting instead to specialized services. As a result, the professionals working in the UBSF should be as close as possible to this type of user, to help support their daily needs, in home visits, in education and health for the population. To demystify disability as a disease, social exclusion and incapacity (WERNECK; FARIA; CAMPOS, 2009).

Even if the disabled person needs more specialized care, this care must be shared, i.e. the user must return to the basic unit for concomitant follow-up (at the UBS and the Specialized Unit), reinforcing the idea not only of social inclusion, but also of including family members in the care. It is essential for humanized, complete and effective care that the needs of people with disabilities are addressed, while understanding and visualizing the needs of their families. This all-encompassing assistance, which goes beyond a single user with individual care, is important to include psychological and social support, guidance for carrying out activities of daily living, offering specialized support in necessary situations, for example, hospitalization or home care.

"Every person with a disability has the right to be cared for in the health services of the Unified Health System [SUS], from Family Health Units to rehabilitation services and hospitals" (FIGUEIREDO, 2011). They have the right to any consultation (medical, dental, nursing), visits from community health workers, basic tests and medicines distributed by the SUS. The UBSF must provide assistance to people with disabilities like any other citizen. In addition, these people are entitled to a specific diagnosis, specialized and rehabilitation services, and to receive instruments and locomotion aids - when necessary, since such equipment complements care, increasing the possibilities of independence and inclusion.

In order to recognize and provide comprehensive care for people with disabilities, health professionals need to be able to approach, naturally and with knowledge, the various aspects that can involve the biopsycho-emotional issues of people with disabilities, namely: Affective issues, sexuality, the exercise of motherhood and fatherhood, topics that are addressed in care and which, in the case of people with disabilities, more precisely with Down's Syndrome, have their own particularities: "If you are a woman and have Down's Syndrome, you can become pregnant and have babies. If you're a man and you have Down's Syndrome, the chances of getting a woman pregnant are very slim, since most of them are sterile (...)" (BRASIL, 2012).

Based on the principles of equality and fairness, the promotion of accessibility and social inclusion involves changing society so that everyone, regardless of group, race, color, creed, nationality, social or economic status, can enjoy a quality life without exclusion. And when it becomes a habit to live with differences without discrimination, inclusion is greater. So that differences are lost in good coexistence, and being "different" becomes "normal" (BRASIL, 2012).

Accessibility aims to enable a wider range of people to gain autonomy and mobility, including those who have had their mobility reduced or have communication or cognitive difficulties. It also concerns the elimination of barriers involving attitudes of prejudice and discrimination, often resulting from a lack of knowledge (on the part of the population and health professionals themselves) of the needs and potential of people with disabilities (BRASIL, 2012).

For truly accessible, universal, comprehensive and equitable care, it is important that the UBS and other health service centers are modified and have physical access, environmental adaptations related to communication, suitable for people with disabilities. Professionals should also be sensitized and trained to welcome and care for people with disabilities. It is also necessary to offer products, instruments, equipment or technologies adapted or specially designed to improve the functionality of people with disabilities or reduced mobility, favoring their personal autonomy (FLEURY S. OUVERNEY, 2013).

The Ministry of Health has been technically and financially encouraging the establishment of reference units for physical, hearing, visual and intellectual rehabilitation, initially in the Federal District and in the states of the Federation. The rehabilitation units aim to develop capacities and abilities in order to promote maximum independence and social participation for people with disabilities. Health care includes not only the monitoring and maintenance of the gains made through rehabilitation and the prevention of disabilities, but also the possibility of receiving and offering the tools necessary for continued rehabilitation. People with disabilities are entitled to the benefits of rehabilitation of their physical, intellectual or sensory state, through specialized assistance and therapeutic workshops, in order to improve their general conditions and their chances of inclusion in school, work and social life (BRASIL, 2012).

Therefore, the universality of care in the Unified Health System means that each and every person, without any kind of discrimination or exclusion, has the right to health care. That health as a right for every citizen goes beyond predefinitions and legislative records, printed or cybernetic files or oratory in political speeches, that it goes from a jargon to a real, developed, effective practice, consistent with each reality and particularity. So that people with disabilities, their families, health service professionals and society as a whole understand that through coexistence between different individuals, an inclusive society is built, strengthening full citizenship, and that this is also a product of the health service.

## 2.4 PLAYFULNESS IN CARING FOR PEOPLE WITH DOWN SYNDROME

It is possible to see that throughout history what has most characterized people with Down syndrome has been intellectual disability. At various historical and cultural moments, people with DS were known by a stigma of incapacity, which still permeates the conceptions of many in contemporary society and makes it difficult for them to be integrated into everyday life.

In ancient times, individuals with Down's Syndrome were considered unfit to join a mainstream school or take part in common social activities, such as work, and this was partly due to the fact that most of the studies published on DS dealt only with the pathological order, and were often pessimistic about their ability to learn and develop, i.e. there was little discussion of the potential that these people have when stimulated (MARTINS, 2002).

However, it has now been discussed, albeit to a lesser extent, in universities, health service centers, educational institutions and legislative centers, that people with DS and other disabilities can be included in the social environment without any damage or delay, as long as they are encouraged to socialize beforehand and the physical environment is consistent with the needs of each citizen - understanding people with disabilities as citizens.

Schwartzman and collaborators (2003) confirm that children with DS go through the same stages of development as a child who does not have the diagnosis, but with some delay, and Martins (2002) emphasizes that among the areas in which each and every child develops their cognition well are the arts, lucidity, musicality, theatricality and play. With this, we have a necessary discussion not about homogenizing the profile of each person in society, but about how interaction between different people can be effective and enjoyable for all.

The term ludic originates from the Latin word *ludus* which, in general terms, refers to games and fun. A ludic activity is also an entertainment activity which gives pleasure and amuses the people involved. The concept of ludic activities is related to ludism, i.e. they are based on games and the act of playing. Playful content is important for learning, cognitive, intellectual, creative, emotional and motivational development, because it instills the notion that learning can be fun (LIMA, 2013).

We understand that play is one of the child's first acts, and that play is an opportunity for development, when the child experiments, discovers, invents, exercises and even checks their abilities. Play stimulates curiosity, initiative and self-confidence, developing language, thinking, concentration and attention. According to Piaget (1975) and Vygostsky (1998), scholars of learning and the child's psyche, through play the child appropriates knowledge that will enable them to act on the environment in which they find themselves, in order to build concepts and acquisitions that in the future will become their basic level of real action and morality.

Mafra (2008) attributed a decisive role to children's play in the evolution of human development processes, such as maturation and learning, opposing many who think that play, games and playful activities are mere pastimes. Playfulness aids and promotes processes of socialization and discovery of the world, so as to stimulate the development of the child's abilities in a natural way, developing motor skills, the mind and creativity, without pressure or fear, but with pleasure.

Based on the idea that play and games are activities that help children's overall development, fostering their self-esteem and the acquisition and learning of new concepts, the pedagogical and school environment should value and encourage work based on playful activities (MAFRA, 2008). However, another environment in which such activities should be present in some way, whether in clinical care practices or in indications, is the health services.

Understanding the active role that play has on the human body, biopsychosocially speaking, health services that use this method provide their users with better self-esteem, self-confidence and autonomy, in order to stimulate co-responsibility in health care. However, it is necessary for professionals to understand that playful actions should be developed as a provocation for meaningful learning and a stimulus for the construction of new knowledge with the development of new skills (GOULAR; LUCCHESI; CHIARI, 2010).

When it comes to the work of health professionals, in addition to the requirement for technical knowledge essential to their area of activity, there is a need for knowledge linked to other areas, including personal skills in dealing and living with the collective, individual and cultural diversity that permeates our society (GOULART; CHIARI, 2007).

Considering that being healthy is not restricted to the absence of illnesses, but rather the admission and evaluation of biopsychosocial aspects; It is not enough for health systems to focus solely on pathological cures from a biologicist point of view; it is essential to restructure health policies and actions to promote health, taking into account the cultural and subjective dimension required by health care, with playful practices being an indication for broader and more equitable care actions (COELHO; ALMEIDA, 2005).

Thus, practices in health services that take into account humanization, comprehensive care of the person, understanding the stage of life they are in, can use playful activities, especially with regard to child development and people with disabilities, "playful actions, games and games for children with intellectual disabilities are primary activities that bring great benefits from a physical, intellectual and social point of view" (MAFRA, 2008).

Since it is proven that playful activities promote growth and biopsychosocial development in human beings, educational institutions, as well as health care institutions, should adopt them as mediators of learning, socialization and activities that help form the critical awareness of each citizen. Since playfulness makes it possible to build a new way of educating and working together in solidarity (MAFRA, 2008).

Contrary to the idea that health care services are limited to biologicist clinical practices, it is possible, through multidisciplinary projects and new methodological approaches (for example, the use of playful practices in health centers), to break the stereotype that health care institutions (basic, medium or high complexity) are a tense, stressful environment, where there are predominantly painful reactions of fear and anguish (MARINELO; JARDIM, 2013). In this way, care becomes humanized, and the person being cared for, including the person with intellectual disabilities, externalizes and expresses their feelings and imagination, so that the playful actions encourage the health service user to be more accepting of undesirable situations, helping them to achieve a better emotional balance and adapting them to face social resistance (MAFRA, 2008).

Playful activities also help to improve the user's (especially children and people with intellectual disabilities) communication with the professionals in the multidisciplinary team, as well as the positive recovery of the trauma or deficit that led the user to seek health services. As well as being used in therapy as an aid to communication between users, professionals and carers, playfulness contributes to improving the practice of health education - facilitating understanding of health prevention and promotion so as to make each user co-responsible for their health care and empower them to assist in health.

It is thought that playful practices, exemplified by therapeutic play, bibliotherapy, art therapy, musicality, theatricality, dynamics, decorative environments, among others, are not limited to the area of pedagogical practice, or to an exclusive health care sector (MARINELO; JARDIM, 2013). Playful activities can and should be developed in the various health care sectors and institutions, at the levels of Basic Care, Medium and High complexity, configuring themselves to each space and demand, in order to further humanize care and not limit it to pathological treatment and cure. Despite the fact that care is structurally divided into levels of care, the common aim is to prevent, protect and promote health (WERNER; SANTOS; TOMAL, 2012).

However, despite the benefits, the implementation of playful activities in today's health care design is not simple, there are a number of difficulties: lack of training for professionals (since their academic training) in the practice of playful activities, lack of funds to purchase and maintain the materials needed for playful activities, the small number of professionals needed to provide comprehensive care to health service users (MARINELO; JARDIM, 2013). It's like a paradox that playful, integrating activities are advocated, but the basic support to carry them out is not provided.

The wide-ranging discourse on play and games allows us to draw a metaphorical parallel between the concept of play and life - the game of life, the game of powers, valuations and exclusions that permeates our society. Huizinga (2000) describes play as older than culture, pointing out a very interesting aspect: that even in its simplest forms, at animal level, play is more than a physiological phenomenon or a psychological reflex, it goes beyond the limits of purely physical or biological activity. It is a *meaningful* function, that is, it contains a certain meaning.

In play there is something "at stake" that transcends the immediate needs of life and gives meaning to action. Every game means something, no matter how you look at it, the mere fact that the game contains meaning implies the presence of a non-material element in its very essence (HUIZINGA, 2000).

There is a divergence between the numerous attempts to define the physiological, biological and even psychological function of play. Some define the origins and foundations of play as the discharge of superabundant vital energy, others as the satisfaction of a certain "imitation instinct", or even as a constituent in preparing young people for the serious tasks that life will later demand of them, such as exercising self-control. There are also theories that consider play to be an "ab-reaction", an escape from harmful impulses, a restorer of the energy expended by a one-sided activity, or "wish fulfillment". One element common to all these hypotheses is that they start from the assumption that play is linked to something other than play itself, that there must be some kind of purpose in it, including, but not limited to, a biological one (HUIZINGA, 2000).

If we see that the game is based on the manipulation of certain images, on a certain "imagination" of reality (in other words, the transformation of reality into images), then our fundamental concern will be to capture the value and meaning of these images and this "imagination". And we are encouraged to think about what imagination or image has been created about the disabled person, about the person with Down's Syndrome, in the social game. Whether in this game of values and recognition of social rights, the particularities of people with disabilities are being respected and considered beyond a sentimentality of pity or charity (HUIZINGA, 2000).

At first glance, when we talk about play in caring for people with Down's Syndrome, we think of play activities exclusively in terms of biologicist clinical care with, at most, multi-professional support. The possible relationship between play and law, justice and jurisprudence seems distant. The whole sphere of law is dominated by the seriousness and vital interests of the individual and society. The etymological foundations of most of the words that express ideas related to law and law are mainly linked to the notions of establishing, indicating and ordering (MARINELO;JARDIM,2013).

All these ideas seem to offer little or no relation to the semantic sphere that gave rise to the ludic terms, and even seem to be opposites. However, the possibility of a kinship between law and play becomes clear as soon as we understand the extent to which the actual practice of law, i.e. the process, is extremely similar to a competition. And whatever the ideal foundations of law may be, there is a premise of struggle, conquest and determination on the part of the social spheres of people with disabilities to demand the full and equal assistance that is theirs by right. This has strengthened social movements which, paradoxically, are fighting for the social inclusion of people with intellectual disabilities and Down's syndrome (CABRAL; FERREIRA, 2013).

Some of the organized civil society movements for people with disabilities intend to break away from the predefinition and definition of a standard of intelligence and intellectual resourcefulness, in which those who don't meet the idealized profile *"are out of the game"* have difficulties entering the social environment, the fields of education, work and even health care - when care is broken down into specializations, classifying who will accompany the health and disease process (CABRAL; FERREIRA, 2013).

Therefore, although the discussion of playful practices is usually focused on the pedagogical level (school institutions), the health care sector can develop such practices with the aim, in addition to health education, of achieving the best motor and intellectual development of people with DS, thus contributing to the improvement of humanized care techniques. This care will be reflected in the social integration of people with DS, so that they will not be at a disadvantage in the "game of life", but in the right.

# 3.RESULTS AND DISCUSSIONS

We understand that nursing, like other professions, is guided by a work process, which is defined as the transformation of an object into a product through the intervention of a human being who uses instruments to do so. Thus, work is something that human beings do with intention and consciousness, with the aim of producing a product or service that has value for human beings themselves (MARX, 1994).

The nursing work process is basically divided into four components (assisting/intervening, teaching/learning, researching, managing), which have their own objects, instruments, methods and products. Although subdivided, there is a common purpose to all the components of the work process, which is to maintain quality of life, promoting and preventing health (SANNA, 2007).

It is necessary to emphasize that the work process is not watertight or carried out by just one of its components. The relationship between assisting/intervening, teaching/learning, researching, managing and articulating, so that these processes sometimes occur simultaneously (HORTA, 1979).

This articulation and simultaneity in the nursing work process makes the profession useful to society and those it serves. Nursing is a process of action, reaction, interaction and transition between individuals and groups in a social system in order to achieve health objectives or adjust to health problems. The products of this process are the result of the combination of political power, social recognition and favorable conditions for operating the work process. In short, despite the understanding by its executors of what the nursing work process is, there are agents who coexist and influence how it is carried out and what is defined as work (HORTA, 1979).

It is clear that there is a need to discuss nursing care with a broad range of contents and contexts, highlighting the instances of professional training, deepening the theory on the part of professionals, returning to the daily work of health services - understanding them as spaces for the political participation of nursing professionals.

Thus, it is important to understand the execution of nursing work based on the system that governs health services - the Unified Health System, in order to get closer to the care strategies used for people with Down's Syndrome, and what aspects interact with the obstacle of truly equitable care; in accordance with the principles and doctrines of universality, integrality, equity, resolubility, decentralization, citizen participation (BRASIL, 1990).

## 3.1 NURSES' KNOWLEDGE OF DOWN SYNDROME

The nursing professional's knowledge of Down's Syndrome helps the person with Down's Syndrome to get along well with their family, as well as society; since this professional acts as a guide to possibilities and choices for a better development process for the person with the disability (NEGRI; LABRONICI; ZAGIONEL, 2003).

*"Basically, during nursing appointments We try to demystify DS as a disease, due to so much prejudice that still exists, we try to socialize the person with the syndrome with their own family, because sometimes the person with the syndrome is much more open to this socialization than the family" (Cuidadosa).*

In this way, other professionals must adopt a positive, open attitude, considering the genetic alterations common to DS not purely as limitations. The actions of health professionals must be in line with the reality of each user, whether they are a person with a disability or not.

Knowing the physical and anatomical characteristics of people with DS is important for monitoring and evaluating their health and disease process. Understanding their particularities and specificities will lead to better care.

*"Knowing that this person with DS can live normally, even depending on specific care" (Capaz).*

*"(...) I even had a suspicion at the CeD once, a suspicion, I never confirmed the diagnosis, but I suspected it because of the characteristics" (Playful).*

Therefore, nurses' understanding of Down's Syndrome empowers them to better recognize the manifest signs of people with DS. Since it is often the nurse who recognizes the syndrome, refers the user to the health service for follow-up and medical assessment and works with the family on the news and the experience of mourning the syndrome.

Sassi (2013) states that mourning and disability are two inseparable terms for parents and family members who are faced with a child/parent whose limitations hinder, delay or prevent them from carrying out tasks that other people can eventually do, and in many cases, "the child with a disability is not compatible with all the dreams that were built up during the parents' long waiting process".

In this time of mourning, Sassi (2013) points out that the work of health professionals is fundamental to stimulating reflection on the internal and external changes that need to happen in parents and family members. In other words, professional help influences internal growth and external support so that parents and family members can develop resources to deal with the reality of the person with a disability, allowing them to visualize the positive aspects of this new relationship (a different relationship from the one they had before). In this way, the participation of this professional helps to build relationships (disabled person - family - society) in a healthy, spontaneous and loving way.

But what can be seen from some of the professionals is that there is a certain fear of exposing their knowledge due to their superficiality about Down's Syndrome

*"Assistance methods are incipient, this public is not so prioritized" (Hiperativa).*

*"(...) there are difficulties in assisting people with DS, mainly because of the different way we would have to treat them, and often professionals in general, not just nurses, have this difficulty, let's say they don't have the specific knowledge for this assistance" (Playful).*

In view of these statements, we are led to question whether the specific knowledge is due to the training offered in the formal spheres or to the interest in seeking to build it through and for the professional's daily experience.

*"And if (a person with DS) came in today, I would provide normal care, like everyone else. I would do the nursing consultation depending on what they needed and I would also make a referral to the specialist doctor, depending on demand" (Alegre).*

*"(...) we don't have any specific work for people with DS, although there are cases in our area, but we've never done any specific work for them. If a person with DS arrived at the UBS, they would have a normal nursing consultation, like everyone else, if they had diabetes or hypertension, we would treat it like a hyperdia consultation, it would be a consultation according to the program that was needed" (Playful).*

This being the case, equitable care is hampered by the lack of knowledge of some professionals, and the dimensions of nursing practice, such as care-education-research, are sometimes restricted to a certain public (by programming care), leaving people with disabilities at the mercy of technological models of health care that massify or represent a mechanistic way of approaching the health process, are sometimes restricted to a certain public (by programming care), leaving people with disabilities at the mercy of techno-healthcare models that massify or represent a mechanistic way of approaching the health-disease process, full of possibilities to be explored, as well as the failure to comply with public policies aimed at people with disabilities, in this case, Down's Syndrome. In this way, the professional reinforces the flexitarian model and the fragmentation of health work, or directs the search for specialized services, with allegations of unpreparedness to provide care for people with DS.

In contrast to the statements made by many professionals, we can see that there is production of information on disability, assistance and legal security for people with disabilities, especially those with Down's Syndrome. An example of this is the creation of the Manual for Health Care for People with Down's Syndrome, which aims to offer instructions to multi professional teams in the different care services. Its content refers to guidelines for clinical diagnosis, identification and treatment of pathologies associated with DS, as well as guidelines for health actions for the various stages of life of users with DS - childhood, adolescence, adulthood and old age (BRASIL, 2012).

## 3.2 APPROACH TO DIVERSITY CARE IN THE (IN)FORMATION OF NURSES.

There is a notorious lack of knowledge on the part of society and many health service professionals about equitable care (which guarantees the right to health for individuals, whether they have a disability or not), so we need to discuss and reflect on this as a factor in ineffective actions in health care and promotion, which indirectly ends up contributing to the stagnation of the care panorama (HIGARASHI; PEDRAZZANI, 2002).

The importance of the work of qualified and informed professionals is increasingly emphasized, in order to assist people with disabilities to include them in society, respecting their rights, knowing their limitations and, above all, their potential, as well as the best way to work on these potentials (HIGARASHI; PEDRAZZANI, 2002). However, what can be understood from the words of some professionals working in health services is that there is a lack of information about assisting people with disabilities, especially those with Down's Syndrome, as well as a lack of appropriation of assistance to diversity in their own professional training.

*"(...) during my training I didn't see, we didn't receive any guidance in the academy about how to assist a person with Down's disease, at least in my training I didn't have any approximation" (Committed).*

*"Because in reality our training doesn't prepare us well for almost anything, there is a holistic training of the world, of the health and disease process, but specifically of certain pathologies it doesn't train us, although there are presentations of some pathologies and syndromes, there is no in-depth discussion, and what is in theory is often dissociated from practice, perhaps if there was a better theoretical approach, perhaps practice today would be different, I would have a better approach to these patients" (Cuidadosa).*

*"(...) there is nothing from the ministry to guide nursing consultations for people with DS" (Playful).*

So, in overview, the training of nursing professionals in health services, especially those working in Primary Care and the Family Health Strategy, leads us to question whether there is compatibility between care and the real needs of the service. In addition to the convenience of some professionals when they hold the health service management body responsible for their own knowledge, when what is necessary and indicated would be the daily search for new knowledge, understanding the diversity that is life, and consequently, the diversity of knowledge that is needed to assist it.

It is true that during academic training there is a construction and adaptation of knowledge and skills that must be implemented by each professional, but there are no closed, exact or watertight ways of constructing knowledge, it requires a continuous search, preparation and reconstruction of learning.

In parallel with the nursing education provided by the Faculty of Nursing (FAEN) of the State University of Rio Grande do Norte (UERN), we can see that the graduate profile, in line with the National Curriculum Guidelines for undergraduate courses, is that of a critical and reflective nurse with the technical, scientific, ethical-political, social and human skills to exercise and coordinate their work process. A nurse capable of (re)constructing knowledge for action in defense of the quality of life, comprehensive health care and the quality of services provided to the population without restricting individuals, that is, the nurse must be able or qualified to provide non-selective care, knowing how to assist people with disabilities or not (UERN, 2014).

At the same time as a general analysis of the curriculum matrix and the appropriation of the syllabus contents of the above-mentioned education unit, we can see that there is little discussion of the social inclusion of people with disabilities, or even health care for people with disabilities; For example, the subject of caring for people with Down's Syndrome is only discussed in the subject Semiology and Semiotechnical Nursing in the Health-Disease Process of Children (coding 0501009-1), which in a peculiar way corroborates the stereotype of infantilization of people with disabilities, of people with DS. It would be important to add this discussion to the other disciplines and components of the curriculum, understanding the breadth of assisting people with disabilities, while not treating this subject punctually (UERN, 2014).

According to Brasil (2001), the profile of the graduate/health professional (nurse and other professionals) must be able to develop actions of prevention, promotion, protection and rehabilitation of health, both on an individual and collective level. This profile must also be identified with a capacity for continuous learning (both in their training and in their professional practice). Thus, health professionals need to learn how to learn and be responsible and committed to their education, as well as to the training/internships of future generations of professionals, providing conditions for mutual benefit between future professionals and service professionals, including stimulating and developing academic/professional mobility.

In addition to the guidelines for training in health, considering the equity that is required for each person in health care, there are other instruments that help to build ongoing knowledge, for example, the Manual and Guidelines for the Care of People with Down Syndrome, made available in printed form to all health regions, as well as accessible to the whole of society through communication networks. These guidelines advise professionals on health care for people with Down's Syndrome throughout their life cycle. They are designed in a practical way, in simple language, and can be used to provide health advice to people with disabilities and their families (BRASIL, 2012).

The production of information on disability and legal security for people with disabilities, especially Down's Syndrome, in the field of health care is thus evident. At the same time, there is a need for each professional to continue their (in)training in order to understand and transform the social inclusion of people with disabilities into a living, pulsating force.

The discussion of assistance for people with disabilities is not something that exists today. It has been a long time since people have been thinking, researching and forming guidelines (including legal ones) about this assistance. An example of this is the Salamanca Declaration (1994), formulated by consensus between several countries and safeguarded by the United Nations Organization, which defines standard rules on equalizing opportunities for people with disabilities, with a focus on state security for their education, and also discusses perspectives on health care. Some of the indications are

*"Parallel and complementary legislative measures should be adopted in the fields of health, social welfare (...). Community rehabilitation should be developed as part of an overall strategy with the support of combined efforts between disabled people, their families and communities and the appropriate education, health and welfare services (...). Coordination between educational authorities and those responsible for health, work and social assistance should be strengthened at all levels in order to promote convergence and complementarity (...)"* (BRASIL, 1994).

So information exists, but you have to look for it. Houaiss (2008) uses the term information as knowledge obtained through research, such as clarification, explanation, indication, communication or information. Referring to health information, we can see the multiple dimensions that can be used to support the health sector itself: in the administration of this sector, in assistance, in action planning, in surveillance, among others (MORAES, 2007). However, many professionals working in health services are resistant to working with this information (both seeking it and producing it), which results in a reductionist approach to programs, without the equity and breadth that is required of health care.

*"(...) because even at university we didn't see this, at least I didn't see DS in my training, I saw it from above, on my own... The biggest obstacle is the very lack of discussion about disability, about inclusion, in my day these discussions didn't exist, I think this has come now, because it's a necessity to discuss this type of assistance" (Playful).*

*"I didn't see anything about DS in my training, at the time I went to university there weren't these discussions that we know exist today, about disability, about DS. What I know today was more from day-to-day life, something I read" (Alegre).*

The care so advocated in health services requires knowledge of the specificities and the most appropriate approaches for each part of the population, in order to guarantee equity and democratization of health care, without losing sight of the individualization of health care (HIGARASHI; PEDRAZZANI, 2002). Continuous training is required for professionals who are already working, as well as for future professionals who are still in training units. When this (in)training is not obtained, aspects of insecurity are generated in professionals, leading to problematic care without continuity and responsibility for care. *"(...) And we're often afraid that we won't be able to cope, so I prefer to refer them straight away" (Cuidadosa).*

*"(...) if there is this information about assisting people with DS, as soon as it arrives at the health units, we have to go and get this information privately, and if there are any normative guidelines, we are not aware of them, and we are often not so prepared for this assistance" (Committed).*

As for the unpreparedness mentioned by the interviewees, Higarashi and Pedrazzani (2002) show that studies converge on the idea of the inability or lack of preparation of health professionals to carry out this practice (of assisting people with disabilities), when professionals are aware of the need for preparation, some individually seek to improve their practice, and others settle for waiting for training from the service coordinator.

By identifying the difficulties and aspects that interact with the failure of care practices for people with disabilities, especially those with DS, the professionals themselves express their need for: specific and continuous preparation (courses, continuing education), theoretical training (the training itself), the need to integrate information between professionals and services, in order to generate multiprofessional and multisectoral care (when, for example, professionals working in a Basic Health Unit link up their services with professionals from the Psychosocial Care Center or other elements of the health care networks and, based on an assessment of the needs presented by the service user, they also link up with highly complex care units).

*"First of all, it's the question of training professionals, so that we can provide better*

*assistance, because I believe that in the area of education this discussion is broad, but in our area the discourse is incipient, we're not even demanded by managers for this assistance" (Empenhada).*

*"(...) academia needs to help build pedagogical teaching mechanisms that can make the student wake up, and that this student leaves the walls of the university for training in the daily life of the service, so that he has a new look, including at the person with Down's Syndrome" (Cuidadosa).*

*"Nobody is born learned, what I can say is that nursing is practically everything, whether it's cardiology, gynecology, pediatrics, in all of them nursing has to have a little knowledge, but for that we are, and we must be trained, I believe that there is no difficulty in doing any service, but first we need to have knowledge and training on how to deal with each situation, with each user we assist" (Carinhosa).*

*"Well, speeches about equitable care also need to be present in professional training, and the university, unfortunately, is still a long way from this. Universities need to build up this knowledge in their students. And we also need to have a permanent education policy in place, to have the resources earmarked for this policy actually being spent for this purpose and not diverted" (Capaz).*

With regard to the insecurity reported, Werneck (1997) refers to the problem of the care provided by these professionals, the need to train human resources in order to promote, in an integrated manner, the qualification of personnel at all levels of training and services, so as to achieve better working conditions and higher productivity rates.

*"(...) we get close to the subject, but in a very superficial way, and so, we individually try to research how people with DS have been monitored and cared for, and it's important for health professionals to look for readings, to keep up to date, and to apply this to their practice, because training in itself, and I believe that no training, gives us a*

*plenitude of knowledge" (Hiperativa).*

*"(...) I remember a training session I attended here in the city, which wasn't even about DS specifically, it was about inclusive care, we discussed disability and we also talked about DS, 95% of what I know, I did the research myself" (Capaz).*

Thus, the incipiency and superficiality of discussions and training about assistance to people with disabilities, people with DS, both at the level of health services and in health training or education. It is necessary to re-evaluate how these services are structured and how professionals understand and care for people with disabilities and Down's Syndrome. Although some of the professionals in practice or even those who have graduated today show superficial knowledge about assisting people with DS, politeness about disability has a historical-social construction, and the expropriation of assisting people with disabilities is not peculiar to current training.

Mantoan (2003) points out that education in Brazil has been structured around segregative welfare models, segmenting people according to their disabilities or abilities, contributing to the education of a person with a disability or the pedagogy of disability taking place in a "world apart", as something extra and not commonplace in education. The author also points out that discussions of special education in our country began in the 19th century, inspired by North American and European models, as a form of isolated action based on purely biological concepts.

## 3.3 NURSES' UNDERSTANDING OF DOWN IN AN INFANTILIZED WAY

In the discussion about people with disabilities, we see a search for inclusion. Including society; a concept that goes beyond sharing a physical space, materials and activities. Thus, the idea of inclusion anticipates the development process of the disabled person and the process of readjusting social reality.

Ciampa (2004) states that human beings are considered products and producers within their historical and social context. Thus, it is only possible to understand human behavior from the relationship established with others. The concept of the disabled person is influenced by the social context, by what they think of themselves and how others understand them.

From this we are urged to reflect on how individuals identified with intellectual disabilities, especially Down's Syndrome, are perceived, understood and cared for in health services, especially in the conception of the nurse working in Primary Care, who most of the time becomes a pioneer in investigating and recognizing the disability, in indicating interdisciplinary care and in working with the family that is mourning the syndrome.

*"(...) the nursing care we provide here is limited, it's practically CeD consultations. And we don't have the conditions, for example, in the CeD to do this consultation as recommended by the ministry because of the demand, which is very high (...)" (Cuidadosa).*

*"I do more of the full CeD, providing guidance, monitoring, checking on breastfeeding, vaccinations, if anything comes up that I can't solve I refer it to the doctor, that's my job. There's not much for us to do in the unit, apart from guidance, because right here we have nothing to follow up. And so, there are professionals who don't even know how to deal with a person with DS, only if it's, for example, a child who does CeD" (Alegre).*

*"(...) at CeD we pay attention to the particularities that children with DS have, remembering that this child's development will take a little longer because of the disability, so we evaluate according to the reality, always giving guidance to parents, calming these family members - because mothers generally always like to compare their children with each other, comparing development and weight - my boy already does this, what about yours?" (Capaz).*

The way in which nurses approach and guide people with DS and their families is fundamental to their inclusion in society. And in the words of some professionals, we can identify an infantilization of people with Down's Syndrome when they refer to the consultation of people with DS only at the CeD, not explaining, if there is any, a follow-up of this service user throughout their life cycle - adolescence, youth, adulthood or old age, when identified by the ESF teams.

It is thought that in addition to classic prejudice, which is characterized by discrimination against what is different (with an idea of distinction or belittlement), another form commonly identified as prejudice in relations with people with intellectual disabilities is the concept of incapacity and incompetence projected onto them (SOUZA, 2007). These conceptions tend to infantilize people with disabilities, making them perform the most basic tasks on the assumption that they won't be able to, which can be seen as disrespecting or omitting rules for supposed "advantages" conditional on disability.

Melo (p.8, [n.d.]) provides basic guidelines for the best development, including social development and autonomy, of people with intellectual disabilities; guiding them to avoid overprotection, whether the person is a child, a young person, an adult or an elderly person, it is important to help them in whatever way is necessary. Young people or adults with intellectual disabilities should not be treated in an infantilized way. "Only treat them like a child if they are a child".

The statements of some professionals can be interpreted as converging in explaining why people with DS are seen in such a way.

*"(...) approaching a child is easier, because we can even work on their socialization, guide the family, and when they are already an adult there is a particularity and even greater care in how to approach them, because sometimes they may not understand" (Hiperativa).*

*"(...) it's difficult for us to get close to them (people with disabilities in the older age groups), if we had approached them earlier, our relationship would certainly have been different, certainly much better" (Cuidadosa).*

Thus, when it comes to assisting children, there is greater ease and mastery of knowledge in care. With regard to the disabled in the older age groups, the professionals speak of insecurity and unpreparedness, referring the difficulty of care to the inability of the young/adult/elderly disabled person to understand health guidelines.

*"I think this discussion needs to be introduced even more at university, in subjects such as children's health, understanding that the way children are approached reflects on their attachment to the health service as adults and their commitment to their own health" (Hiperativa).*

The perspective of assisting the person with DS during childhood or as an eternal child is corroborated by the professional's speech when they expose the need to discuss the theme of this assistance in training in order to fix this discussion in the discipline that builds knowledge about children, for example Semiology and Semiotechnique of Nursing in the Health-Disease Process of Children (0501009-1. CONSEPE, Resolution No. 05/2010). As if the health of adolescents, women, men and the elderly did not apply to people with Down's Syndrome or were not seen in their corresponding stage of life (UERN, 2010).

Brasil (2012) states that health care in DS should be singularized to the life cycle. With a view to maintaining health and better developing the potential of people with DS, the aim is to improve their quality of life and social integration.

Therefore, we need to pay attention to nursing care that provides opportunities to prescribe care to promote, protect and recover children's health, carrying out educational activities to improve the growth and development of both the child and their caregivers. Nursing care that understands adolescence as a stage of life whose main causes of morbidity and mortality are external causes (violence, traffic accidents, drug addiction, unwanted pregnancies, among others), so that nurses can identify vulnerability and design their work around actions that reduce the problems considered. Systematic nursing care is consistent with the particularities of each user, whether they are women, men or the elderly, revealing itself in an equitable way that is consistent with realities (GENIOLE et al, 2011).

Therefore, in carrying out their care, nurses need to know, understand and form coherent care for each stage of life. Understanding and treating the service user in accordance with their life cycle, whether they have a disability or not. Brasil (2012) emphasizes the importance of effective communication between professionals, people with DS and their families; the importance of multi-professional and interdisciplinary follow-up, with guidance on exams, specialized treatments and encouragement for the social inclusion of people with DS; and the provision of unique health care in life-cycle care models when health service professionals focus on promoting healthy lifestyles in the family nucleus.

## 3.4 ATTENTION TO PEOPLE WITH DOWN SYNDROME IN HEALTH CARE NETWORKS.

According to Brasil (2010), Brazilian health care has been organized around organizational arrangements of health agencies and services of different technological densities which, integrated through technical, logistical and management support systems, seek to guarantee comprehensive health care; these arrangements are known as Health Care Networks (RAS).

The implementation of the RAS directs health services towards greater efficiency in health production, improvements in the efficiency of the management of the health system at each level of care, in order to strengthen the articulation between basic, secondary and tertiary care, contributing to the advancement of the process of making the SUS effective (MENDES, 2011).

Extending the right to assistance and care to people with disabilities, the Care Network for People with Disabilities was promulgated within the scope of the Unified Health System by Ordinance No. 793/2012, with a view to corroborating the principles and doctrines of the SUS and making public through yet another legislative document the right to comprehensive and equitable health care for people with disabilities.

The Care Network for People with Disabilities aims to increase access and improve care for people with disabilities; to promote the linking of these people and their families with the points of care, whether at a basic level or more complex, in order to guarantee the articulation and integration of health care points and services (BRASIL, 2012d).

Although there are recommended forms of health care for people with disabilities, including people with Down's Syndrome, there is a dichotomy in the fulfillment of these care guidelines, when some professionals consider and adopt these guidelines in their work process; others are unaware of them, and consequently don't apply any guidelines in their service; and there are still those who are aware of the guidelines for better care for people with DS, whose equitable care is a necessity in their area of care, and yet they don't apply them.

Thus, paraphrasing the statements of the nurses who took part in the research with the incisions of the Care Network for People with Disabilities within the scope of the Unified Health System:

*"also working with the family in assisting people with Down's Syndrome (...) providing the necessary support for these people, both in terms of physical structure with the material needed for assistance and in terms of personnel, professionals trained to provide this assistance" (Hiperativa).*

We see convergence when the recommendation is to support and guide family members and companions of people with disabilities, as stated in Article 16, item IV, of Ordinance 793, as well as to promote humanized, equitable care centered on the needs of health service users, whether they have disabilities or not, as clearly stated in Article 2, item V, of the same ordinance (Brasil, 2012d).

*"It's important to work on the issue of prejudice, the importance of placing or encouraging people with DS in the social environment so that their families understand that people with disabilities should be active and participate in society" (Hiperativa).*

In this way, assistance respects and encourages the fulfillment of human rights, in order to guarantee autonomy, independence and freedom for people with disabilities to be co-participants in their health and disease process; promoting respect for differences and acceptance of people with disabilities, confronting stigmas and prejudices as portrayed in Art. 2, items I and III, of Ordinance 793, (Brazil, 2012d).

In contrast to the statements of professionals who agree with the guidelines of the Care Network for People with Disabilities, there are professionals who are unaware of any indication of care and assistance for people with disabilities, especially those with DS.

*"I don't know if there really is any specific guidance for assisting people with Down's disease, but I think there is, and what usually happens is that care guidelines, standards, don't arrive here at the unit, we can't access them, what arrives goes to the secretariat and stays there, there's no transfer" (Capaz).*

*"No, I don't even know if it exists, nothing has arrived here yet, nothing to guide us on how to care for people with DS. Only if there's been something like this for doctors, because there hasn't been anything like this for nurses yet" (Alegre).*

*"If it exists, it hasn't reached the unit, and I don't think it's reached primary care, but the Ministry of Health is always producing standards of care, but I'm not aware of any specific ones for DS. I've taken part in events at the city or municipal health secretariat on a wide variety of subjects, but those specific to DS haven't appeared here yet" (Carinhosa).*

So, even though there are instructions on how to care for people with Down's Syndrome, most professionals are not aware of them, and this lack of knowledge affects care that should guarantee comprehensive care, open access and assistance with the specificities inherent and indispensable to the care of people with disabilities. Werneck (1997) states that a society for all should be aware of the diversity of the human race, and therefore structure itself to meet the needs of every citizen, from majorities to minorities, from the privileged to the marginalized.

Care for people with disabilities must exist to ensure access to health services, good communication, understanding and execution of appropriate clinical management. Finally, because it materializes as the realization of equity, since there are guidelines for care, as well as instruments and guiding devices for intervention, promotion and protection of the health of people with disabilities, so that health professionals are able to give up the act of blaming or finding something that "justifies" the non-existence of care for people with disabilities, that is, something that conceals their professional disinterest.

*"(...) I don't even know if there are any guidelines for this type of care, and if there are, we haven't yet reached them. But I think that the limit comes from the professionals themselves, who perhaps aren't well prepared for this type of care, and there's this difficulty in getting close to this reality, so it's necessary for professionals to adapt to each type of care, assisting both the person with DS and the family who need differentiated care" (Cuidadosa).*

That said, care for people with disabilities, especially those with DS, is a commitment of the health service, from management to professionals working in primary care.

When we refer to the Network of Care for People with Disabilities, we realize the co-responsibility of managers for the care of other care professionals. Article 2, items X, XI and XII of Ordinance 793, indicates the promotion of permanent education strategies taking into account the care needs of people with disabilities; it is necessary to develop a logic of equitable care for people with disabilities (physical, hearing, intellectual, visual, ostomy and multiple disabilities) having as its central axis the construction of a singular therapeutic project by a multi-professional team; to make progress in carrying out clinical and epidemiological research, taking it as an aid to providing a more qualified service and performing with the social integration of people with disabilities and their rehabilitation technologies (Brasil, 2012d ).

*"We should do an active search to find out how many people with Down's are in our*

*area, in what conditions they live, and then start thinking about strategies to help them" (Committed).*

*"(...) I think it's important to do an active search, to find out if there are any people with DS and how many there are, it's important, and with this result we would do work for this group, first the active search, then we would plan how we would care for this public. And we'd even work with other institutions like the church, UEI, these things (...) I don't know of any UBS that works with or assists these people, together with other support institutions" (Playful).*

It would be good if professionals working in Primary Care and the Family Health Strategy were interested in seeking out and getting to know people with disabilities living in the area covered by the Basic Health Unit where they work, in order to understand their needs and design coherent care for them.

Sassaki (1997) points out that the process by which the general systems of society, such as the physical environment, transportation, social and health services, education, work and culture, must be made accessible to all. This includes the removal of physical barriers and attitudinal barriers that prevent people with disabilities from participating fully in all areas (primarily health care), thus enabling them to achieve a quality of life common to all other people and to participate actively in society.

This point is reinforced by Decree 5.296/04, which in its completeness provides basic criteria for promoting accessibility for people with disabilities, by referring to accessibility in architectural and urban constructions, social housing, cultural goods, information and collective communication (Brasil, 2004b).

Decree 7.611/11 also discusses the promotion of accessibility for people with disabilities, now in the school environment, providing for specialized educational assistance (AEE). The objectives of this assistance, in Article 3 and items I to IV, are the promotion of conditions for access, participation and learning in regular education, with a guarantee of support services according to the individual needs of the students; the transversal guarantee of special education actions in regular education; the development of didactic and pedagogical resources that eliminate barriers in the teaching and learning process; and ensuring conditions for the continuity of studies at other levels, stages and modalities of education. Article 7 also states that the Ministry of Education must monitor access to school for people with disabilities, in partnership with the Ministry of Health and other management bodies, in order to ensure more comprehensive care (Brasil, 2011).

In the problematization of reality, even though the discussion on accessibility and inclusion is gaining ground in the legislature and in education, health care services are not yet fully integrated into these debates and constructions.

*"(...) We don't carry out any activities for this group here, even though we know it exists in our territory, and these people don't come to the unit, I think because they know that there are few professionals here who are prepared to help them, and I think they go straight to the specialized service" (Empenhada).*

*"(...) I know that there are users in my area, if I'm not mistaken there are a couple of them, but so far they haven't come to me, they're like they don't need my assistance, because we visit them, but that's what we're wanted for, but so far their families haven't come to us" (Carinhosa).*

It is understood that some of the professionals working in primary care have the minimum knowledge necessary to assist people with disabilities, or to investigate how this assistance should be given; however, this attention, interest and concern for users with disabilities does not materialize as a priority. We realize that there is a need to rethink the duty of the health service to reach its users; the system that governs health care is not unidirectional, in the sense that only the user should seek the service. But it is bidirectional, i.e. of dual interest and responsibility, when the health service represented by its professionals must go to its user (BRASIL, 2013).

*"(...) Due to the high demand, we haven't been able to associate the care of people with disabilities very well with the routine practices of the service, but at the level of of social assistance, health education activities are always implemented for this public. (...) Thus, we do not have and have not been trained to assist these people (...) In addition to our overload of service that does not allow us to take a differentiated look at people with DS, with disabilities, the prejudice that exists in the community, even among the professionals themselves, may be the cause of many of these people not seeking out the unit" (Committed).*

Among the aspects that interact with the failure to provide equitable and inclusive care for people with disabilities, especially those with DS, we have noticed the unpreparedness of professionals to assist people with Down's Syndrome, most of the time due to a lack or incipient knowledge of the subject; as well as a high demand, when the number of users who come to the service does not match the capacity of the reduced number of professionals to assist them; as well as the social prejudice that still exists about Down's Syndrome, which means that many family members don't decide to go to the health service, or when necessary they go to secondary and specialized care, without exposing the person with DS to the community in which they live. In fact, these aspects need to be worked on in an attempt to minimize and eliminate them from the production of health services.

*"We need to improve the care network, articulate the services even more, treat primary care as the real gateway to the health system" (...) always trying to associate primary care with other structures such as CRAS, NASF, in short, working as multi-professional teams, as we should" (Hiperativa).*

And when there is coordination between the services, there is a positive response to the care, as can be seen in the words that exemplify an experience of caring for a person with DS:

*"(...) we tried to work together with other sectors, forming an intersectoral approach. (...) From then on, we continued the follow-up with the other professionals: cardiologist, physiotherapist, speech therapist, we started these follow-ups in a rehabilitation unit, a unit that had a multi-professional team, and the mother was also assisted, with consultations with the psychologist.(...) So we made contact with the pediatric referrals, so that there would be a broad and articulated follow-up between the health sectors and services. And I, as a nurse, didn't shirk my responsibility for care and continued to accompany that child with DS and his jam ilia" (*Hyperactive).

In this way, co-responsibility is understood with health care, rearranging its service to the particularities of each health service user.

*"(...) And depending on the degree of DS, the child will have a later development, and here we always refer them to a more specialized care, a pediatrician, for this shared monitoring, because we know that this child in particular needs monitoring by a cardiologist of specialized doctors due to their different anatomy, and there is a need for multiprofessional monitoring. And so, we try to do this, with the integrality of the system, within a network, this child goes through and we can accompany and stimulate them for development' both the child and the family, because support for the family is important" (Capaz).*

Professionals are still discussing a view of people with DS that is still based on "degrees" or factors of severity, rather than thinking of this human being in terms of their biopsychosocial dimensions, a way that has already been emphasized by the World Health Organization itself. It therefore advocates the importance of shared and continuous care, which goes beyond curative methods, with extensive interventions and multi-professional attention to the health of people with Down's Syndrome.

*"(...) And SD then leaves everything to APAE? But is that right? Wouldn't it be better for APAE to work with the UBS to monitor people with DS? And APAE itself should be referring them to us - because in these referral centers they have socialization, but they socialize with people just like them, and the other part, socialization with other people,*

*with the other side, with the community, we (the unit) should also be accompanying them, but we know very little about their lives" (Cuidadosa).*

This statement reveals the need to recognize the gaps presented by the service as a whole, as well as the lack of understanding about the Care Networks. In this way, the production of health services reflects the notion that prevailed in previous decades of the 20th century, that the care and education of people with disabilities and/or special educational needs was restricted to specific institutions. This clearly exclusionary model elucidates the stereotypes created by society, whether for massification, standardization according to criteria of beauty, functionality or the performance of socio-historically constructed roles.

In this way, fostering care beyond the health unit, with follow-up in line with the socializing and specialized pedagogical unit, will also involve the exchange of experiences between professionals from each unit. This coordination should be extended to other pedagogical institutions which are not necessarily specialized but which share the care of people with DS.

*"(...) "We don't have the means to work on medical issues during the consultation period, nor do we have links with other services, such as the UEI next to our unit, so that we can work on these playful issues, but there is often a lack of participation, interaction, partnerships and availability on the part of the professionals, we know that the ESF is made up of multi-professionals, but unfortunately historically the nurse is the one who "carries the ESF", This partnership with the UEI can happen through any professional (ACS, doctor, dentist, social worker) but it seems that the nurse needs to be at the forefront, to drive things forward, or things don't happen, we nurses already have so many obligations, that sometimes we forget the good influence that these partnerships have, and so we don't prioritize and consequently we don't execute" (Cuidadosa).*

Some nurses' explanations for not practicing complementary activities in the care of people with disabilities and for not articulating the health service with other services are often meticulousness, overload in the services, low professional self-esteem or not treating the articulated care of people with DS as a priority. And the difficulty of coordination is not just between the different services.

But for Mantoan (2006), viewing people with disabilities from the point of view of including them in society must be totally and radically effective, above all by respecting and valuing differences. This means that inclusion also implies a change in the understanding and conduct of professionals (including health professionals), in order to propose a social organization and care system that takes everyone's needs into account. Inclusion has no exceptions, it respects the rhythm of each person's life and is based on human potential, as opposed to a society that disables and reinforces the impediments of people with disabilities. There is a need for inclusive care (which values and guides inclusion) as an attempt to reverse the (still persistent) exclusionary framework of today's society.

*"(...) But there is a difficulty in the very articulation between the care sectors, we as primary care gain the reliability of the family, but when we refer them to other services they are often lacking. As a result, the link becomes frayed due to successive disappointments with the service. As far as it depends on us as primary care professionals, there is a need for greater and better knowledge, but that's not all, there comes a time when we need other dimensions that we don't have" (Capaz).*

So, despite the material and care shortages, it is necessary to clarify all the difficulties for the user and their family, so that the inadequacy of the service is not seen purely as incompetence on the part of the professional, which leads to discrediting the work of that professional. But when the user understands the reason for the lack of quality in health care, they become an endorser in the fight to guarantee their rights, the right to health.

*"And that the managers in particular had an idea of what the DS is and what needs to be done, and in my opinion it is the managers themselves who need the most training. (...) that the professionals have constant training, updates, that the service network*

*works, that we are able to have comprehensive care, with references and counter-references, that this family has support within this network, and that we have the personal and material conditions to work" (Capaz).*

The importance of caring for a person with DS in a shared and continuous way, in a health care network, should be considered by health service managers, professionals and users. So that health care becomes a shared responsibility and not a transferred one.

## 4.FINAL CONSIDERATIONS

Through this research, it was possible to broaden our understanding of the problem of the development of care strategies for people with intellectual disabilities, specifically Down's Syndrome, which were developed by nurses working in Primary Health Care, while we observed a lack of individual and collective actions related to health promotion, disease prevention and rehabilitation of users with disabilities.

There was little interest on the part of some professionals in seeking better care strategies for people with DS and their families, in contrast to the qualification and reorientation of health practices currently indicated by the Expanded Clinic model, as advocated by the Ministry of Health at this level of care.

It was also possible to confirm the assumptions initially raised in the essays of this work, when the identification of the aspects that interact to hinder equitable care for this clientele are recognized (including by the research participants themselves) as: lack of an academic approach to caring for people with disabilities and/or DS; lack of ongoing training for professionals working in primary care (in relation to caring for people with disabilities); lack of human resources needed to meet the dynamics of the service, i.e. there is a lack of service to the number of professionals working in Primary Care, which contrasts with non-singular and disjointed care at all levels of care, with real transfers of care responsibilities and no sharing of these.

Among the population of nurses selected for the survey, the need for contextualization in terms of the variables of community, society, political and social contingencies and inclusion was apparent in their care. This need was present both in the understanding and implementation of care strategies for people with DS and in terms of the actions deemed important for transforming the current care framework. The target audience felt uncomfortable with the co-responsibility of providing better care for people with disabilities and improving it.

The objective of this study was achieved when we learned about the nursing activities aimed at assisting people with Down's Syndrome in Primary Care, so that the necessary equity in care was not identified.

Furthermore, the discourses on the production of care often highlighted the insecurity of the majority of professionals, the superficiality of their knowledge about caring for people with disabilities, often treating clients with DS in a childish way, when there are already guidelines for caring for people with Down's Syndrome that take into account the particularities of people with DS during their life cycle.

Thus, care for users with DS must meet the proposals of health promotion, prevention of possible complications and inclusion of users with DS in society, guiding and/or applying playful activities in care that enhance the approach of this clientele.

Among the practical implications and contributions provided by this study, we can identify the judgment of the interviewees regarding the improvement of professional preparation, which is reflected in greater safety for the exercise of care activities and, consequently, an improvement in the quality and effectiveness of the care provided to clients with DS, in a way that encouraged practicing professionals and the scientific community (with a representation of nursing professors and students) to approach assistance tools (including playful instruments) for cognitive stimulation and the inclusion of people with DS in society, since it is impossible to reverse the genetic/chromosomal condition that determines DS.

With the breadth of the subject discussed here, new data is suggested to be worked on, in other words, a direction for future studies can be developed in the perspective of discussing the articulation between different levels of care for people with disabilities; conceptions of people with DS and their families about multiprofessional care - potentialities and challenges; nursing care as an inclusive tool; among other optics and conceptions that this work stimulates to be debated.

## REFERENCES


BRAZIL, Ministry of Health. Technical Nucleus of the National Humanization Policy. **HumanizaSUS**: the expanded clinic. 1ª ed. Brasilia: Ministry of Health, 2004a.

BRAZIL, Ministry of Social Action. Civil House - Legal Affairs Sub-Cabinet; **Decree 5.296/04**, Brasilia: Ministry of Social Action, 2004b. Available at: http://www.planalto.gov.br/ccivil_03/_ato2004-2006/2004/decreto/d5296.htm. Accessed November 20, 2015.

BRAZIL, Ministry of Health; Health Care Secretariat. **Guidelines for the Care of People with Down Syndrome**. Led. Brasilia : Ministry of Health, 2012a.

BRAZIL, Ministry of Social Action. Casa Civil - Subchefia de Assuntos Juridicos; **Decreto 7.611**, Brasilia: Ministerio da Agao Social, 2011. Available at: http://www. planalto. gov.br/ccivil_03/_Ato2011- 2014/2011/Decreto/D7611.htm#art1. Accessed November 20, 2015.

BRAZIL, Ministry of Health. Secretariat of Health Care. **Health care for people with disabilities in the Unified Health System - SUS** , Department of Strategic Programmatic Actions. Led. Brasilia : Ministry of Health, 2009.

BRAZIL, Ministry of Health. **Health care for people with Sown Syndrome,** Department of Strategic Programmatic Actions Serie F. Brasilia: Ministry of Health, 2012b. Available at: http://bvsms.saude.gov.br/bvs/publicacoes/cuidados_saude_pessoas_sindrome_dow n.pdf.

BRAZIL, Ministry of Health, National Health Care Secretariat. **ABC do SUS: doutrina e principios**. ed.1 p. 1-10. Brasilia-DF, 1990.

BRAZIL, Ministry of Social Action. National Coordination for the Integration of People with Disabilities. **Salamanca Declaration and line of action on special educational needs**. Brasilia: MAS/ CORDE, 1994.

BRAZIL. Ministry of Health. Health Care Secretariat. Department of Strategic Programmatic Actions. **Manual de Atengao a Saude da Pessoa com Sindrome de Down.** Brasilia: Ministry of Health, 2012c.

BRAZIL. Ministry of Health. Health Care Secretariat. **National Health Promotion Policy**. Brasilia, DF, 2006a.

BRAZIL. Ministry of Health. Health Care Secretariat. Department of Strategic Programmatic Actions. **Manual de legislagao em saude da pessoa com deficiência**. ed.1 p.368. Brasilia-DF, 2006b.

BRAZIL - Ministry of Health. **Redefines Home Care within the scope of the Unified Health System (SUS). Ordinance No. 963**, of MAY 27, 2013. Available at:http://bvsms.saude.gov.br/bvs/saudelegis/gm/2013/prt0963_27_05_2 013.html Accessed: April 19, 2015.

BRAZIL, Ministry of Health; Minister's Office. **Establishes guidelines for the organization of the Health Care Network within the scope of the Unified Health System (SUS). Ordinance No. 4.279**, of December 30, 2010.

BRAZIL, Ministry of Health. **Care Network for People with Disabilities within the scope of the Unified Health System.** Ordinance No. 793, of April 24, 2012d.

BRAZIL, Ministry of Education. **National Curriculum Guidelines for Undergraduate Nursing Courses**. RESOLUQAO CNE/CES N° 3, of November 7, 2001.

BRAZIL, National Health Council. **Resolution No. 466 of December 12, 2012**. Regulating research with human beings, 240ª Ordinary Meeting. Available at: http://bvsms.saude.gov.br/bvs/saudelegis/cns/2013/res0466_12_12_2012.html. Accessed: April 09, 2014.

BARDIN, Laurence. **Content Analysis.** Lisbon: Edigoes 70, 2010.

BRITO, Tabatta Renata Pereira. Playful practices in everyday nursing care Pediatrics. **Escola Anna Nery Rev. Enfermagem**, v.13, n. 4, p. 802-808, 2009.

Bento, A. **How to do a literature review:** Theoretical and practical considerations. Revista JA (Associagao Academica da Universidade da Madeira), n. 65, v.7 , p. 42-44, 2012. ISSN: 1647-8975. Available at: http ://www3. uma.pt/bento/Repositorio/Revisaodaliteratura.pdf. Accessed September 20, 2014.

BERNARDES, L. C. G. et al. People with disabilities and public policies in Brazil: bioethical reflections. **Ciencia e Saude Coletiva**, Sao Paulo, v. 14, n. 1, p. 31-38, 2009.

CIAMPA, A. da C. **PSICOLOGIA SOCIAL:** o homem em movimento. Sao Paulo: Brasiliense, 2004

COSCRATO, G.; PINA, J. C.; MELO, D. F. de. The use of playful activities in health education: an integrative literature review. **Acta Paulista de Enfermagem**, Sao Paulo, v.23, n. 2, p. 257-263, 2010.

CAMPOS, G. W. **Saude Paideia**. 3ª ed. Sao Paulo: Hucitec, 2007.

COELHO M.T.A.D ; ALMEIDA F. N. **Concepgoes populares de normalidade e sau- de mental no litoral norte da Bahia**, Brasil. Cad Saude Publica;v. 2,1 n.6, p. 1726-36, 2005

CARNEIRO, M. S. C. **Adults with Down syndrome**: Mental disability as a social production. Campinas, SP: Papirus, 2008.

CABRAL A.V.; FERREIRA G. **Social Movements and the Protagonism of People with Disabilities**. SER Social, Brasilia, v. 15, n. 32, p. 93-116, jan./jun. 2013 Available at :http://periodicos.unb.br/index.php/SER_Social/article/viewFile/9599/7136,

Accessed: January 7, 2015.

DAPS, Health Care Secretariat. **Information series on Down's Syndrome**: for healthcare professionals. 3ª ed. Brasilia, DF, [n.d.].

DIAS S. V.; OLIVEIRA M. C. S. L. Deficiencia Intelectual na Perspectiva Historico-Cultural: Contribuigoes ao Estudo do Desenvolvimento Adulto. **Rev. Bras. Ed. Esp.**, Marilia, v. 19, n.2, p. 169-182, 2013.

DEZOTTI , M. C. **Individual with Down Syndrome: history, legislation and identity**.2011. 167f. Dissertation (Master's in Special Education) - Faculty of Education, University of Sao Paulo, Sao Paulo, 2011

FLEURY S. OUVERNEY A. M. **Health Policy: a Social Policy**, 2013. Available at: http://www.escoladesaude.pr.gov.br/arquivos/File/TEXTO_1_POLITICA_D E_HEALTH _POLITICA_SOCIAL.pdf. Accessed on: January 07, 2015.

FARIAS N.; BUCHALLA C. M. The International Classification of Functionality, Disability and Health of the World Health Organization: Concepts, Uses and Perspectives **Rev Bras Epidemiol** v.8, n.2, p.187-93, 2005. Available at: http://www.scielosp.org/pdf/rbepid/v8n2/11.pdf Accessed October 24, 2014.

FIGUEIREDO E. N. **A Estrategia Saude da Familia na Atengao Basica do SUS.** Open University System of the Unified Health System - UNA-SUS/UNIFESP, 1st ed. Federal University of Sao Paulo, 2011.

FIDALGO, A. **Semiotica Geral**. University of Beira de Interior, Covilha, Rio de Janeiro, 1999;Online Library of Communication Sciences. Available at: http://www.bocc.ubi.pt/pag/fidalgo-antonio-semiotica-geral.pdf. Accessed: April 2, 2015.

GIARETTA, A.; GHIORZI, A. R. The act of eating and people with Down syndrome. **Revista Brasileira de Enfermagem**, Brasilia, v. 62, n. 3, p. 480-484,

May-June 2009.

GENIOLE L.A. I. [et al.] **Nursing care by life cycles.** Campo Grande. ed. UFMS : Fiocruz Unidade Cerrado Pantanal. v.8 p. 240, 2011. Available at: http ://www.portalsaude.ufms .br/manager/titan. php?target=openFile&fileld=351 Accessed: April 14, 2015.

GOULART B.N.G.; LUCCHESI M. C.; CHIARI B. M. a Unidade Basica de Saude como espago ludico para educagao e promoga da saúde infantil - relato de experiencia. **ev. Bras. Crescimento Desenvolvimento Hum**. v.20 n.3, p.757761, 2010.

GOULART B.N.G, CHIARI B M. Integrality and Humanization: general perspectives and contributions for reflection. **Rev Soc Bras Fonoaudiol** v.12 n.4. p.335-340. 2007.

HEIDEGGER, M. **On Humanism**. Translated by Emmanuel Carneiro Leao. 2.ed. Rio de Janeiro: Tempo Brasileiro, 1995, p.94-95.

HIGARASHI H.I. , PEDRAZZANI C. J. The professional nurse and children with disabilities. **Revista Ciencia, Cuidado e Saude.** Maringa, v. 1 n. 1 p. 37-44. 2002.

HOUAISS, A. **Dicionario Houaiss da Lingua Portuguesa**. Rio de Janeiro: Objetiva, 2008. Available at: www.houaiss.uol.com.br/busca.jhtm

HORTA, V. A. **Nursing process**. Collaboration with Brigitta E. P. Castellanos - Sao Paulo: EPU, p.99, 1979.

HUIZINGA, J. **Homo Ludens**. Sao Paulo- SP, Ed. Perspectiva S.S, v.4, ed.4, p. 3-162, 2000.

INTERDONATO G.C ; GREGUOL M;
Promoting the health of people with disabilities: a systematic review.

**HU Revista**, Juiz de Fora, v. 37, n. 3, p. 369-375, 2012.

BRAZILIAN INSTITUTE FOR THE RIGHTS OF PEOPLE WITH DISABILITIES - IBDD
**Social inclusion of people with disabilities: measures that make a difference** - Rio de Janeiro: IBDD, 2008, p. 312. ed.1.

LIMA B.A. S. **BRINCAR NA EDUCAGAO INFANTIL:** O ludico como estrategia educativa. 2013, 64f. Monograph (completion of Pedagogy course) Faculty of Education, University of Brasilia, Brasilia.
Available at:
http://bdm.unb.br/bitstream/10483/4938/1/2013_BrunaAlessandraSilvaLima. pdf
Accessed: October 26, 2014.

LUIZ, F. M. R. **Experiencias de familiares de criangas com Sindrome de Down no processo de inclusao na rede regular de ensino.** Dissertation for the Ribeirao Preto School of Nursing, Sao Paulo, p. 116, 2009. Available at: file:///C:/Users/Rhianna/Downloads/FlaviaMendoncaRosaLuiz%20(1).pdf. Accessed November 25, 2014.

PAULA. L.A. **Etica e Educagao especial**: uma reflexao sobre a cidadania do portador de deficiencia mental. Master's dissertation in education. Rio de Janeiro, UERJ, 1994.

LEITE B.L. ; GALVAO I. **The education of a savage: The** pedagogical experiences of Jean Itard. Sao Paulo: Cortez, 2000.

LOPEZ M.M. **El Proyecto Roma: una experiencia de educacion en valores**. Malaga: Aljibe, 2003.

MENDES E. V. **Health care networks**. Brasilia: Pan American Health Organization. ed.2° p.549, 2011. Available at: http://www.conass.org.br/pdf/Redes_de_Atencao.pdf Accessed: April 14, 2015.

MARX K. **Capital**. 14ª ed. Rio de Janeiro (RJ): Bertrand; 1994.

MELO F.R.L.V. **Interactions with people with disabilities:** some basic guidelines. Federal University of Rio Grande do Norte, Natal, RN. p.1-9. [n.d.]. Available: www.sistemas.ufrn.br. Accessed April 4, 2015.

MORAES, I. H. S. GOMEZ, M. N. G. Information and informatics in health: a contemporary kaleidoscope of health. **Ciencia & Saude Coletiva**, Rio de Janeiro, v. 12, n. 3, p. 553-565, 2007.

MANTOAN, M. E. **The time and turn of inclusive education.** Education and the family
- Disabilities: diversity is part of life. Sao Paulo, v.1, p.42-45, 2003.

MANTOAN, Maria Teresa Egler. **School inclusion: what is it? Why? How to do it?** v.1 ed.2, Sao Paulo: Moderna, 2006.

MELERO, M. L. **Construendo una escuela sin exclusiones:** una forma de trabajar en el aula con proyectos de invertigacion. M'lada, Aljibe, 2004.

MINAYO, M C. de S.; GOMES, Suely Ferreira Deslandes Romeu. **Social research:** teoria, metodo e criatividade. 28ª ed. Rio de Janeiro: Vozes, 2009.

MALTA, D. C. Lista de causas de mortes evitaveis por intervengoes do Sistema Unico de Saude do Brasil. **Revista Epidemiologia e Servigos de Saude do SUS**. v. 16, n. 4,

p. 233-244. dec. 2007.

MARTINS, L. A. R. A **inclusao escolar do portador da sindrome de Down: o que pensam** os **educadores?** Natal: EDUFRN, 2002.

MAFRA S.R.C. O **Ludico e o Desenvolvimento da Crianga Deficiente Intelectual.** State Department of Education, Directorate of Educational Policies and Programs Educational Development Program . 1st edition, 2008.

MARINELO, G. S.; JARDIM, D. P. Playful strategies in pediatric patient care: applicability to the surgical environment. **Rev. SOBECC**, Sao Paulo. apr./jun. 2013; v.8 n.2 p. 57-66.

MELO, G. L. V. FARIA, V.F. **People with disabilities: conquering rights, building citizenship.** Teresina : SEID (Secretaria Estadual para a Inclusao da Pessoa com Deficiencia) p.64 ed. 1 ,2009. Available at: http://www.seid.pi.gov.br/diversos/cartilha1.pdf. Accessed: February 13, 2015.

NEGRI M.D.; LABRONICI L.M.; ZAGONEL I.P.S.; Inclusive nursing care for people with Down's Syndrome from the perspective of Paterson and Zderad. **Rev Bras Enferm,** Brasilia (DF), v. 56n.6 p. 678-682,2003.
Available at: http://www.scielo.br/pdf/reben/v56n6/a18v56n6.pdf. Accessed: February 14, 2015.

World Health Organization, WHO. **International Classification of Functioning, Disability and Health.** Translated by A. Leitao. Lisbon, 2004.
Available at: http://www.inr.pt/uploads/docs/cif/CIF_port_%202004.pdf.
Accessed October 24, 2014.

PIAGET, J. **The formation of symbols in children:** imitation, play and dream, image and representation. [translation by Alvaro Cabral, 1975]. 2ª ed. Rio de Janeiro: Zahar, 1975.

PACHECO M. V. P. C. Esquirol and the emergence of contemporary psychiatry. **Rev. Latinoam. Psicop**. n.2, v. 6, p.152-157, 2003. Available at: http://www.fundamentalpsychopathology.org/uploads/files/revistas/volume06/n2/es quirol_e_o_surgimento_da_psiquiatria_contemporanea.pdf. Accessed October 26, 2014.

RIZZINI, I.; MENEZES, C.D. **Children and adolescents with mental disabilities in Brazil:** an overview of the literature and demographic data. Rio de Janeiro: CIESPI/

PUC-Rio, 2010.

ROSSI, C. F. F; ROSSI T. M.F. People with intellectual disabilities: schooling policies. In: **VI COLOQUIO INTERNACIONAL- EDUCAGAO E COMTEMPORANEIDADE**, 2012, Sao Cristovao-SE. Educonse,2012, p. 1 to 14. Available at: http://educonse.com.br/2012/eixo_11/PDF/21.pdf Accessed on: February 03, 2015.

SOARES, M.V. B.. Citizenship and Human Rights. In: CARVALHO, Jose Sergio (Org.). **Educagao, Cidadania e Direitos Humanos**. p. 56-65. Petropolis, RJ: Vozes, 2004.

STAKE, R. E. **Qualitative research**: studying how things work. Penso, Porto Alegre, p. 78 - 263, 2011.

SASSAKI R. K.; XAVIER M.A. **INTERNATIONAL DECLARATION ON MONTREAL ON INCLUSION** - International Congress " Inclusive Society" ; Montreal, 2001. Available at: http://portal.mec.gov.br/seesp/arquivos/pdf/dec_inclu.pdf, Accessed on: December 08, 2014.

SASSAKI, R. K.. Disability terminology in the age of inclusion. **Revista Nacional de Reabilitagao**, ano 5, n° 24, jan./feb. 2002a, pp. 6-9

SANTIAGO, M.L. **Intellectual inhibition in psychoanalysis**. Rio de Janeiro: Jorge Zahar, 2005. E-book. Available at: http://books.google.com.br/books?id=RnBdvY1DrBwC&printsec=frontcover&hl= en-BR#v=onepage&q&f=false. Accessed on: 23.Oct.2014

SILVA, N. L. P. DESSEN M. **A. Down's Syndrome: etiology, characterization and impact on the family Interagao em Psicologia**, n. 6 v. 2 p. 167-176, 2002. Available at: http://ojs.c3sl.ufpr.br/ojs/index.php/psicologia/article/viewFile/3304/2648- Accessed: October 6, 2014

SCHWARTZMAN, J.S. ***Sindrome de Down.*** 2.ed. Sao Paulo: Memnon- Mackenzie, 2003. 324p.

SANNA C.M. The work processes in Nursing. **Rev Bras Enfermagem**, Brasilia, v.2 p. 221-4, 2007. Available at: http://www.scielo.br/pdf/reben/v60n2/a17v60n2.pdf. Accessed: February 14, 2015.

SOUZA. D. P. **School inclusion and mental disability:** teachers' views and the process of subject formation. In: 15th Congress of Scientific Initiation, 2007. Methodist University of Piracicaba, Sao Paulo, p.1-4. Available at: http: //www.unimep .br/phpg/mostraacademica/anais/5mostra/ 1/148.pdf Accessed: April 2, 2015.

SASSI,F. **The impact of childhood disability on parents and the process of recognizing this reality through the help provided by teams of health professionals.** In: Psicologia.PT.O portal dos pisicologos. TL0319. 2013. Available at: http://www.psicologia.pt/artigos/textos/TL0319.pdf. Accessed: May 09, 2015.

UERN. Higher Education, Research and Extension Council. **Resolution No. 05/2010-CONSEPE, of February 10, 2010. Regulations for undergraduate courses at UERN.** State University of Rio Grande do Norte, Mossoro, February 10, 2010.

. Rio Grande do Norte State University. Faculty of Nursing. **Course Pedagogical Project. Bachelor's and Licentiate's Degree in Nursing.** Mossoro, RN, 2014.

VIANA, A. C. de L.; FONTERRADA, M. T. de O. **Musicalization as a means of intervention in the development of children with down syndrome - a case study. In: XXI Congress of Scientific Initiation of UNESP, Sao Jose do Rio Preto 2011, Proceedings of the Event. P.** 05170 - 05173. ISBN: 978-8588792-08-1. Available at: http://prope.unesp.br/xxi_cic/27_35387787873.pdf. Accessed on: August 19, 2012.

VYGOTSKY, L.S. **The Social Formation of the Mind** . Sao Paulo : Martins Fontes, 1998.

VYGOTSKY, L.S. **Selected Works:** V Fundamentals of defectology. Madrid: Visor Distribuciones, 1997.

WERNECK M. A. F., FARIA H.P.; CAMPOS K. F. C., **Protocols for health care and service organization.** Belo Horizonte: Nescon

UFMG- Editora Coopmed, 2009.

WERNECK, C. **Ninguem mais vai ser bonzinho, na sociedade inclusiva**. Rio de Janeiro: WVA, 1997. 314p.

WERNER, R. C.; SANTOS, E. F.;TOMAL, T. A. **O LUDICO E A INFORMAÇÃO: A EXPERIÊNCIA DA DRAMATIZACAO NAS ATIVIDADES DE EDUCAGAO EM SAÚDE NO HOSPITAL REGIONAL DE PONTA GROSSA. – Expanded Abstract. In: XX Congresso Internacional Rede Unida, Rio de Janeiro, May 6-9, 2012,** Annals of the Event. n.1, 2012. ISSN: **14143283.** Available: http://www.redeunida.org.br/congresso2012/anais-do-congresso. Accessed on: August 19, 2014.

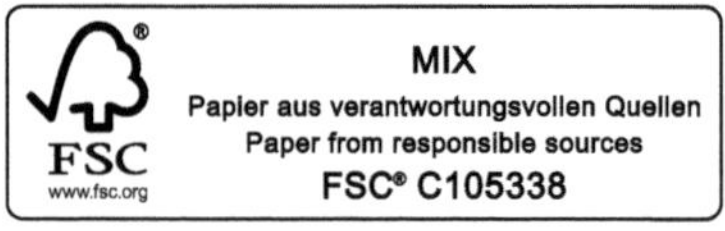


Printed by Books on Demand GmbH, Norderstedt / Germany